# Harriet

*To Kym*
*love from*
*Harriet Devine*
*May 2006*

# Being
# George Devine's
# Daughter

**Barkus Books**

First published in Great Britain in 2006
by Barkus Books
41 The Chase
London SW4 ONP

A CIP catalogue record for this book is available
from the British Library.

ISBN: 09546136-1-9


*Art direction, design and coordination*

Sophie Jump


Printed and bound in Great Britain by
Diggory Press
Three Rivers,
Minions, Liskeard,
Cornwall, PL14 5LE, UK

*For William, Sophie, Oli, Jaz, George, Ben and Cai*

# Contents

# Illustrations

# Acknowledgments

This book would not have been possible without a generous award from the John Hodgson Theatre Research Trust to Sophie Jump, for her research on the illustrations.

I would also like to thank the photographers Roger Mayne and Michael Seymour, who kindly allowed me to include their work at a much reduced rate.

My greatest debt of gratitude is to Donald Howarth, who has generously and enthusiastically encouraged me as well as providing invaluable practical help. Many other people have helped greatly by reading the manuscript at various stages and making useful suggestions: I would particularly like to thank Bill Gaskill, Peter Gill, John Goodwin and Liz Bhushan for various kinds of encouragement and input. Thanks also go to friends who supplied photographs: David Cregan, George Goetschius, Donald Howarth, Alan Mennie, Catherine Mulholland, and Teresa Smith. I am grateful to Edge Hill College for their continued support, and I have benefitted greatly from a Leverhulme Research Fellowship which has enabled me to complete the final stages of this project.

# 1

One day a few years ago I found a large collection of letters from my father to my mother: they had been in the cupboard for a long time but I had never read them, and had in fact forgotten that they were there. There were a great many of them, and I got through them all in the course of a weekend. They told me many things I had never known before.

My father writes to my mother from India:

*25 December.*

*In other words, my precious treasure, it is Christmas day. One year ago, 365 days, I was in easy reach of your loving arms and, to our intense pleasure and excitement, we bumped our Harriet into existence on Larry and Vivien's divan. Or so we like to think, and so we will continue. Last night, Christmas eve, I remembered so well all the details of our arrival at that little house, the tree and the lights, and how we broke the electric light fitting! What a contrast today, and yet I can have sworn so often that I <u>felt</u> you thinking about me when I have lain back in chair or in bed, closed my eyes, and conjured you up before me. It is a cruel fate that our daughter should spend her first Christmas thus, but who knows what the next will be?*

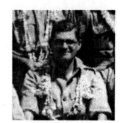

George in the army in India

It's unusual for people to know so much of the detail of their own conception. I know not only the time, the place and the circumstances, but also the mood — 'if only she knew what fun she was to conceive' as my father wrote in another letter. Traditionally children find it impossible, unthinkable, shocking, to imagine their parents in bed together. But the thought of these two people, not in the first flush of youth, still so absorbed in each other after ten years together gives me a warm sense of security, a pleasurable satisfaction to know that my conception was so definitively right for all concerned. I feel it must have been auspicious.

The story of the meeting of my parents is a story I have always known, and one which has always seemed to me to be both romantic and fortuitous. My mother, Sophie Harris, was born in 1900. Her sister Margaret, who was always called Percy, was four years younger. They had a fairly conventional middle-class upbringing in Kent, but their mother was artistic and passed her talent on to her daughters. At art school in London they met a talented young woman of Irish extraction, Elizabeth (Liz) Montgomery. By the end of the 1920s, the three had decided to form a business partnership: the collective name they were to use was Motley. They desperately wanted to design for the theatre, but they had no contacts and no idea how to begin. Meanwhile they were going as often as they could to see the Shakespeare productions at the Old Vic Theatre. Sitting in the gallery with their note-pads, they would make rough sketches of the actors in costume which they would then work up into formal water-colour paintings and sell to the cast for 10/6d. They most admired John Gielgud, who, still only in his twenties, was already regarded as a hugely talented Shakespearean actor. Gielgud bought a number of their sketches, and an acquaintance developed. Over the next few years this gradually grew into a friendship, and in 1930 he invited them to design two costumes for a production of *Much Ado about Nothing* at the Old Vic. The success of these led him, at the end of the following year, to make a much more ambitious suggestion. He had been invited by the president of the Oxford University Dramatic Society (the OUDS) to direct his first production, *Romeo and Juliet*, which was to be performed in early 1932. He would be glad to do it, he said, but he would like to invite his friends the Motleys – 'these three very clever girls' – to design the costumes. The president of the OUDS said no, initially at least. 'We always have our costumes designed by members of the OUDS'. But Gielgud insisted, bringing down some of the girls' sketches for him to see, and he finally

agreed. The president's name was George Devine, and he was to be my father.

The OUDS *Romeo and Juliet* was a highly significant production. Two well-known London actresses, Peggy Ashcroft and Edith Evans, were invited to make guest appearances as Juliet and the Nurse, and when the production opened on 9 February it was greeted by the *Daily Telegraph* as the OUDS' 'best balanced and most satisfying performance of recent years'. For Gielgud it was the beginning of a successful second career as a director, and it gave the Motleys the long-desired break

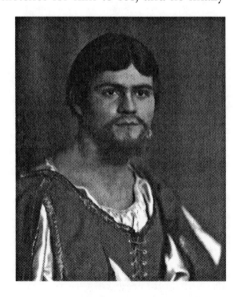

*George as Mercutio in* Romeo and Juliet

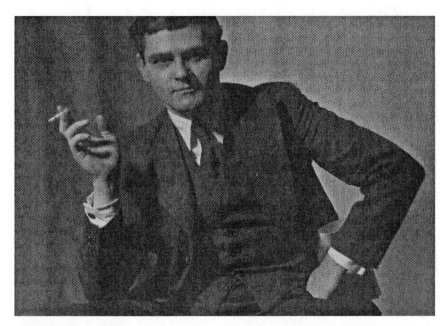

*George in the early 1930s*

which led to their becoming some of the most celebrated theatre designers of their era. Also it certainly played a large part in leading George to abandon his history degree just one term before finals, to move to London and to embark on a professional theatre career. But above all, as far as I am concerned, without it I might well not have existed at all, since it brought about a meeting between my parents. I don't know exactly where George first met the Motleys: perhaps it was in his little rented cottage in Bath Place, which is now an upmarket restaurant. My mother was thirty one, my father only just turned twenty one, but by all accounts the attraction between them was instantaneous and they seem to have started a love affair almost at once.

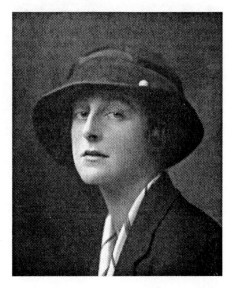

It is strange and exciting to me to think of these people as they

*Sophie in the early 1930s*

4

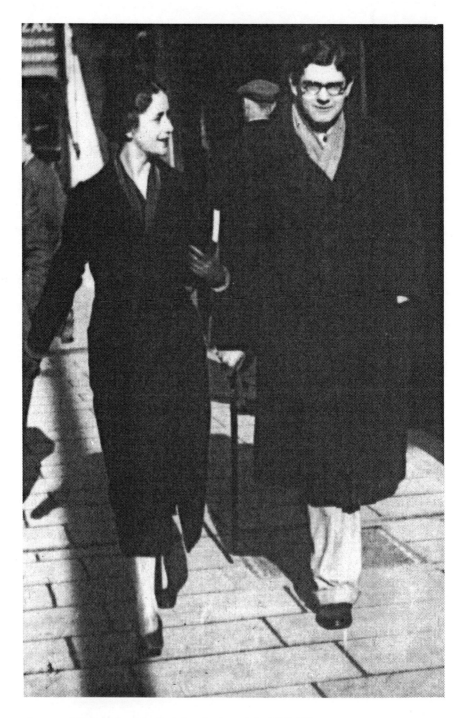

*George and Peggy Ashcroft in Oxford at the time of the OUDS* Hassan were then, much younger than I am now. George was the age of the students I now teach, Sophie more or less the same age as my own Sophie, who never met her grandmother but has also become a theatre designer. I have always wondered how conscious they were of the ten-year gap between their ages. Percy told me that it didn't matter to them when they first met, that it only became a problem later. I'm sure that is true in one sense, but it would be foolish to think that they weren't at least aware of it at the time. Did Sophie, who lied about her age all through my childhood, start lying about it straight away? When George wrote to her many years later, during the war, 'I don't know how old you are, my darling, and I don't want to know', was he being simply disingenuous, or perhaps just tactful? In any case for him, when they first met, she must have seemed wildly exciting – an older woman, beautiful, experienced, generous. For her, after a series of unsatisfactory, empty-headed young men about town, this big, dark, intelligent, funny, moody boy must have been a revelation.

Though he was born in England, George was not English at all. His father was half Irish, half Greek, and his mother Irish Canadian, and he played up his foreign looks, appearing on the streets of Oxford in a huge black overcoat and carrying a cane. Gielgud described him at this time as 'rather ungainly and gross. Very greasy, spotty and unattractive', though he went on to say that 'he had great humour, great charm; and he was immediately very intelligent' , and another contemporary, the actor Anthony Quayle, called him 'portly, his voice…harsh, and his face…verging on the sallow'. But these are men's judgements, and despite his overweight frame, his un-English sallowness and his grating voice George seems always to have been attractive to women: there's a rumour that he had a brief affair with the exquisite young Peggy Ashcroft, probably the year before *Romeo and Juliet*, when she came to Oxford to appear with him in James Elroy Flecker's *Hassan*. In any case, according to Percy, 'George was delightful – intelligent, funny, enormously charming', and Sophie fell in love with him immediately. She had been in love before, had certainly had lovers, the dashing young men with moustaches who appear in our nineteen-twenties family photos. But she had never, surely, had one who was quite like George.

My parents had been together for over seven years when they married in October 1939. In the autumn of 1940, George went for an army medical. He had always believed that his heart was in some way faulty and so he and Sophie were sure he would be turned down. Thus, when he walked in through the door beaming, she thought she knew what to expect. Instead, he waved a piece of paper at her and cried, 'I've been passed –A1!'.

Separated from my mother during his army training in various parts of England, George wrote her many letters. Sophie joined the Land

Army, but stayed in it for less than a year before returning to London. I believe this was owing to the intervention of the theatre manager Binkie Beaumont, who gave her a supervisory job and managed to argue that it was an essential one for the continuance of the London theatre. She and my father met as often as his leaves would permit. They had one particularly enjoyable weekend at the Peacock in Derby ('where every concession is made to the sensual taste' as George rather tantalisingly put it in a letter), but by far the most pleasurable time they spent was the Christmas leave when they were invited to join the Oliviers near Winchester. Larry had joined the

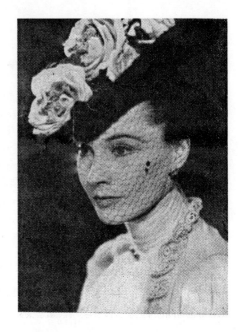

*Vivien Leigh in* The Doctor's Dilemma

Fleet Air Arm and was in training at Worthy Down, and Vivien was touring in a production of *The Doctor's Dilemma* for which Sophie had designed her costumes. They had rented a bungalow at Headborne Worthy, near the airfield where Larry was training, and had invited my parents down for Christmas. Presumably they went there by train, and presumably Larry met them in his 'pride and joy, my Invicta car, with its chromium entrails bursting through the bonnet'. Evidently everyone had a good time – Vivien described the holiday in a letter afterwards as having been 'hilarious and not very restful'. I am not sure how long my parents stayed with them, but it was long enough, evidently, for my mother to become pregnant.

I think they did intend to have a child. I rather gather from reading my father's letters that there had been some kind of consultation with a specialist, and indeed my mother used to tell a story about having been told that she would never be able to conceive. The story was that several months later, hugely pregnant, she had been having tea at the Ritz and had spotted the consultant over the other side of the room. She liked to tell how she had got up and walked over to his table, and then, without saying a word, walked slowly round and round, making sure that he took in every detail of her condition.

Certainly they were pleased and excited to find that a child was on the way. There were the usual anxieties about whether she would get through to the end of the pregnancy ('we can always do it again', my father wrote encouragingly), and the nuisance of morning sickness which George rather irritatingly suggested was all psychosomatic. My mother found a suitably nest-like home in Surbiton, called Little Dell, where George was able to come and visit her during his leaves. But the following June, with Sophie five months into her pregnancy, George's period of training finally came to an end and he embarked for the East. He wrote her a long and loving letter on the eve of his departure:

> *You will probably have gathered, my Soph, that I am about to depart: indeed by the time you receive this letter, I will have left for an unknown port and an unknown destination. I know this will cause you a pang, my honey, because you are, thank God, not made of the metal of the soldier's wife, but I beg you, with all my fervour, to be of good heart, because I know, as sure as I know that I love you, that we will meet again some day, and that it may not be so very long. This war seems long and dramatic, but it isn't really: we have had some very gay and delightful experiences, we have completed our physical love by conceiving a child, and I pray it will be a strong and good one, to be a sign of the bond between us. I face the future with great hope: I am in better health than I have ever been since you have known me, and this will affect my work after the racket is over. We have many good friends, many kind people around us, and we have nothing to fear. All that seems to me so much more important than the blasted war, that I contemplate my voyage as an adventure, and one to be enjoyed. Should misfortune befall me, cherish our child, but never change from being the Sophie I love, and married. Always be my Sophie, not anyone else's, like the Careys, or the Motleys Sophie; I think the world of you, my dearest one, and bless you eternally for your love and faith. So I clutch a small packet of your letters, and expensively equipped in the best style, set out to conquer, with few regrets, a good deal of humility, but much hope in the future, our future, whatever, however, whenever.*
>
> *I cannot end this letter — it has no end, because I think my love for you has none and that is all I can say. I embrace you with all my heart and soul until we see each other again. What a lovely day that will be.*
> G.

So George set off, as he said, for an unknown destination. It is impossible that Sophie did not suffer, but her friend Jill Furse, facing a similar situation shortly afterwards, wrote an encouraging letter to her own departing husband urging him to bear up, and using my mother as an icon of bravery: 'We ought to think how Sophie and others are able to endure it'.

By the time I was born, on 18 September, my father had arrived in India, where he was to spend a tedious eighteen months, mainly in Mysore, waiting for a Japanese invasion that failed to materialise. Worse than the boredom was the fact that there were huge problems with the mail. After the spate of telegrams, airletters, postcards and letters that greeted my birth a huge hiccup occurred, and over the whole period of my first Christmas my mother went for two months without so much as a word from my father. She knew he was alive, as she would have heard if he was not, but the strain was severe, and was exacerbated by the fact that

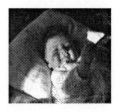

*Me at four months old*

she was suffering from severe post-natal depression. Her cousin Josephine Leeper remembers seeing her at the time looking 'very tense and nervy' and 'confiding in my mother that she kept wanting to throw the baby out of the window'. The culmination of all this was that she ended up being admitted to hospital – the Park Hospital in Oxford, for some reason – on 6 March, and staying there for six weeks, paid for by the generosity of Binkie Beaumont. Meanwhile, I was apparently left in the care of a nurse at the home of friends in Kingston-on-Thames.

Of course I don't remember any of this. I have always known about it vaguely, but my father's anxious letters, written after the mail back-log had cleared, bring the story into sharp focus. One of the worst aspects of war-time separations must have been the delayed conveyance of news. At the best of times mail to and from India was taking at least ten days, and often it took as much as two months, ensuring that all news was old news before it arrived.

All George's delayed Christmas and New Year letters finally arrived in a lump. They were forwarded on to the Park Hospital in March and early April, and I hope they did my mother good and speeded her recovery. I think they must have cheered her. He was a most assiduous letter writer, often sending a letter every two or three days, and no-one could, I believe, have asked for more loving, tender, interesting letters than those he wrote from India. There are so many – more than two hundred – and a whole book could probably be written just about them. They tell of his fascination with India, the people, the landscape and the wildlife, his exasperation with the bureaucracy of army life, his occasional forays to colonial clubs where the conversation was crashingly boring and the women dowdily dressed and chronically adulterous ('I am retiring more and more into my shell and prefer to sit in my hut and read in the evenings'). Like all soldiers' letters they speak of his longing for home: for talks about the theatre with his friends and colleagues, but above all for the good times he remembers with Sophie, 'in your dressing-gown at Mecklenburgh Square', 'in your Steibel coat at a first night', 'among the bluebells at Clobbs Farm': 'I practically live on memory, and a vivid imagination is a great consolation'. The tenderness and the passion seemed to increase as the years dragged on with no visible end to the dreariness of separation.

And as the months went by, they spoke of his fascination with the daughter he had never seen; 'the thought of you and the child keeps me going'. Sophie sent descriptions, testimonials from others, anecdotes and finally photos which helped to bring to life this baby whose arrival had been so strange to her father: soon after my birth he wrote, rather sadly, that he felt:

> *very unhappy in the sense that I cannot fully realise it out here: it seems like a story about someone else, in which I am interested, but I can't somehow really attach it to myself.*

The letters written during the period of over three years that elapsed before he saw me in person are full of wishes for my future and my well-being. He hoped I would not be '<u>too</u> serious'; that I would get to love and understand the countryside as well as Sophie did; that I would love music, and pictures, and books; that I would turn out to be 'an attractive, nice girl...so that we can be friends with her'. He feared that they would hate my boyfriends and think no-one good enough for me. Receiving a particularly appealing set of photos of me aged about two, he wrote to thank her for sending

> *such perfect pictures of HSD. She is the most exquisite and delicious creature I must say and looks as wicked and seductive as hell. I really think I shall be passionately in love with her.*

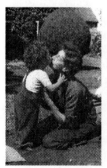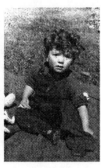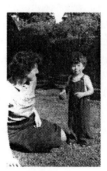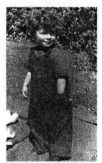

*Aged about two, with Sophie in the garden at Terry's Field*

If the first eighteen months of my father's Asian posting were boring, the second eighteen, spent in Burma, were hugely stressful. It was probably as a result of the Burma campaign that his completely black hair turned snow white. Not that his regiment was involved in a great deal of fighting: they seemed to spend most of their time trekking through the jungle after the Japanese, and trekking back again to where they started from. On one such expedition, in the midst of impenetrable jungle, George lost his signet ring and, happening to be the same area a few months later, offered a cash prize to anyone who managed to find it. To his astonishment, one of the regular soldiers turned up with it, having apparently discovered it caught on a thorn among some overgrown vegetation. In Burma his letters became less frequent and certainly a good deal more despondent, although as the end of the war came into sight there was an upsurge of hope for the future.

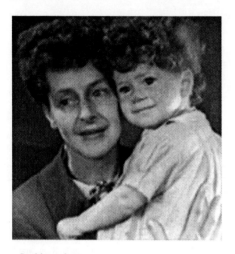

*Sophie and me*

My mother and I meanwhile had moved out to Downe, in Kent. We lived at Terry's Field, a house that belonged to Liz Montgomery's mother Buzz, who became a surrogate granny to me. Our life at Terry's Field seems to me to have been a happy and peaceful one. My mother, now fully recovered, took great delight in me and in my development. Buzz was on hand to baby-sit if Sophie happened to be working, something she never entirely stopped doing, and even though we were rather too close to Biggin Hill airfield to be completely free from the war and the bombing, all in all it was the kind of contented country life that both my parents wished for me to have. But nothing can ever stay the same. As the end of the war approached, and my father began making plans for his return to England, my parents' letters became full of concerns about where they should live. Sophie suggested renting her childhood home, the White House at Hayes in Kent, but George was worried about being too close to her bourgeois relations. They were in the midst of discussing the possibility of flats in London when two things happened: Buzz died, causing Liz to put Terry's Field on the market, and my mother's Uncle Wilfred died, leaving her and Percy a quite substantial sum of money – enough to buy a house: 'I love you all the more now you are rich!', George wrote gleefully. So, as my father prepared to leave the far East and sail for England, my mother had found a large Georgian house in Edwardes Square, just off Kensington High Street, and was busily decorating and furnishing it for my father's return.

# 2

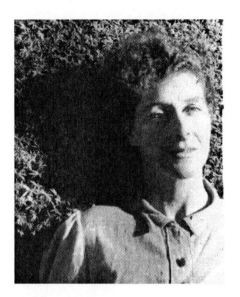

*Sophie at Terry's Field*

My first memories are disconnected episodes, like a series of moving snapshots, and only contain my mother. The very first seems to have been when I was very tiny, less than two years old. We were at our house in Kent, Terry's Field. My mother wanted to go to the bathroom and I wanted to go with her, but she went too fast for me, though I followed as quickly as I could. She disappeared through the door and I clutched at the doorframe, but she didn't know I was there and the door closed on my fingers. I screamed very loudly. My fingers were squashed flat but after the pain went away it was a relief to discover that the fingers had come back to being fat and round again.

Tiny though I was when we were living in Kent, I knew that there was a war going on. Because we were so near to Biggin Hill airfield there were often air raids. We would hear the sirens and we would have to hide underneath a huge iron table in the downstairs dining room. This, my mother explained, was because the Germans might drop a bomb on the house and the table would keep us safe. I did not very much enjoy being under the table even though she tried to make a game of it, with plenty of cushions to sit on and books to read. I realise now that I didn't enjoy it because my mother and Buzz, who we lived with, were frightened, though they never said so. One night a bomb actually dropped in a field not far from the house. Next day I went for a walk with Buzz to look for the place where it had fallen. There was a huge hole in the middle of the field with a mass of twisted metal sitting in the middle of it, looking extremely scary and menacing.

Around the time of my third birthday we went to stay with some friends of my mother's called the Humphries. They had children who were a few years older than I was, and I expect my mother thought it would be good for me to encounter them, since as far as I remember I had never played with anyone of my own age. But the experience turned out not to be a very good one. All I remember of it was that at lunchtime I was sitting at a large table next to my mother, and something was happening which seemed to me to be very strange. A big girl was actually on top of the table, walking up and down, in among the dishes of food and jugs of water, clumping in her big shoes. Round the outside of the table were sitting a great many people, mostly adults, including her mother and father. She was singing loudly and soon she picked up her fork and started to comb her hair with it even though it had mashed potato on it. No one said anything to her, though my mother put her arm round me and squeezed me tight. Afterwards she told me that her friends, the girl's mother and father, did not believe in telling their children what to do. They thought they would grow up to be better people because of this. I didn't really understand this but I was glad she was with me as I found the big girl and her twin brother, who must have been at least two or three years older than I was, very large and loud and frightening.

Another day we went to visit a friend who lived in a big house with a large garden. It was a beautiful bright summer day. The garden had a huge green lawn, which I thought was the most enormous fun to run about on. There were some places on the lawn which were different from the rest, little squares that were very bright green and shiny looking. So as I ran, I decided to try jumping onto one of them. But when I did, I got a shock. Suddenly I was not on the lawn any more, but standing in a little pond of

water which came right up to my waist. I howled very loudly, then I looked to see what my mother was doing. I hoped she would be sorry for me and come and rescue me, but what I saw was her and her friend doubled up with laughter. I cried even louder, because I knew they were laughing at me.

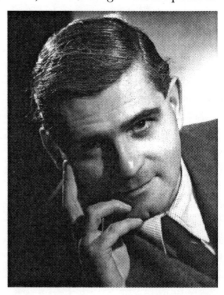

My mother tried hard to make me aware of the existence of the father I had never seen. I suppose many mothers at this time had the same problem. She kept a photo of him in a bakelite frame, which we would look at together every day. George, informed of this practice by letter, was extremely dubious

*The absent father*

about it:

> *don't force the poor mite to look at photos of me! She'll get a complex and 'Dad dad' will be a sort of monster in a brown frame who <u>has</u> to be looked at daily. I should hate it if I were her.*

Undoubtedly he was rather astute in this. Despite the fact that Sophie told me that he would love me very much when he came home, I was not sure how I would feel about him. He had little reality for me, though sometimes he sent me presents from India, and, as I got a bit older, letters for my mother to read to me, which are now sadly lost. Aged about two, I seem to have asked if he could send me 'a sweet little dolly from Burma', and he found one 'which is pretty horrid, but I don't suppose she will mind much'. This apparently took a long time to arrive, and when it did it was 'not up to expectations'. He sent me some shells to play with, and a little necklace also made of shells with a thin string that broke so that my mother had to thread it up again. One time when he was stationed near a convent school, he had some white cotton table mats embroidered for me by the girls at the school: HARRIET, in large red letters.

All those early years I knew nothing but the country. Terry's Field was a wonderful place to live. There was a big garden, and the house sat in the middle of fields, a little way outside the village. Sometimes we went for walks along the side of the golf course, where there were woods, and I would run onto the golf course and into the sandy bunkers, which I liked very much — the sand was beautifully pale and soft. Life was peaceful and rural. But then suddenly it was explained to me that we couldn't stay there any more. Buzz got ill and died, and the house had to be sold. Everything in our lives was going to change. My father was coming home from the war, and we were going to move to a big house in London, 32 Edwardes Square, in Kensington. My mother explained that the square was like a huge garden in front of the house with grass and trees and flowers, and that children could play there. This was presented to me as being almost as good as living in the country but when we moved in I was very disappointed. The square was much dirtier than the country and not so green, and it was all shut in, with high railings all around the outside. Some of the children who lived in the houses round the outside really did get shut in; there were big iron gates that locked, and their mothers would put them inside in the mornings and leave them there, which undoubtedly felt rather like being in prison. At all times of the day there were children hanging on the gates calling out, 'Mummy — come and let me out! Mummy, I want to come out!' I was fortunately too little to be shut in the square but I didn't much like the idea. When I was a bit older and had got used to living in London I came to like it in there very much: it was full of flowers that smelled wonderful, and bushes you could play hide and seek in, and, in the spring, double-cherry trees in full blossom, under which I would lie for hours, gazing up at the blue sky intersected by black branches and huge clumps of white or pink flowers.

Our new house seemed rather dark and, to me, rather frightening. There were black iron railings outside and a gate. If you looked down outside the front door you would see a place called the area, which was always rather gloomy and damp. Looking out onto the area was the kitchen window, and inside the kitchen was Ivy Luker, who was the cook. She had been my mother's Uncle Wilfred's cook, but when he died Sophie not only inherited the money that she used to buy Edwardes Square, she inherited Ivy Luker as well.

While we were waiting for my father to come back we went for a seaside holiday to Margate, and Ivy Luker came too. I had never seen the sea before and I found it a bit overpowering at first, but I liked the sand, which was pale and soft, like the sand on the golf course, except that there was much more of it. Right down by the sea, though, it got dark and wet and squishy, more like mud. One day we were sitting down near the sea in our bathing costumes and Ivy was squidging the sand between her toes. I thought it looked disgusting, so I said, 'Messy old Ivy!' My mother laughed a lot, but I got the feeling that Ivy didn't think it was all that funny. She was a rather gruff elderly woman who had probably not had much contact with small children, having lived and worked in a bachelor household for most of her life. So she was not especially good with me, but there was one thing she did to make me laugh, which was to push her tongue forward and lift up her false teeth on it and make them jiggle about. And when I asked her how old she was she would say, 'As old as my tongue and a little older than my teeth'. Then I would think about her false teeth and wonder how old they were. When I cried she would say, 'Cheer up for Chatham, Dover's in sight'. I never did find out what that was supposed to mean.

It was soon after we got back from our holiday that the time arrived when my father was due to come back from the war. I was not at all sure what I felt about this total stranger coming to join in with our life, but I could see that my mother was very excited. The day before he was due to arrive she made the house unusually clean and then she started on herself. She put curlers in her hair and she had bought some thick creamy white stuff which, I was rather surprised to see, she smeared all over her face. She told me it was supposed to make her look pretty but I thought she looked very odd, and rather like a ghost. When I said this she laughed and said she would be taking it off in the morning before my father arrived. She went to bed very early, soon after me, so that she would be rested when he came next day. But then quite soon, before we were even asleep, the doorbell rang. I heard her get up and as soon as she had gone downstairs I got up too. I was in the hall in time to see her opening the front door. A big man was standing on the doorstep — I couldn't see him very well because it was dark and the street lights were behind him. He was wearing an overcoat and he had cases and bags. He was saying something about trains and times — he was my father, come home a day early. I could see that my mother felt bad because of the curlers in her hair and the white stuff on her face but he didn't seem to mind. Soon they were kissing and hugging and crying, which I thought was strange.

Thinking about it now I really feel for my mother. She was by this time in her mid-forties, and had suffered a great deal during my father's absence. I don't think she ever ceased to be beautiful, but her face was even then quite lined and her hair, once thick and golden, was by this time wispily curly and light brown. It had been four years since my father left for India, and she must have greatly feared that he would think she had aged and lost her looks. If he did, though, it did not seem to make any difference to how he felt about her. In fact he appeared to me to be altogether too fond of her, and, even worse, she was altogether too fond of him. I suffered terribly from this: before he came her whole life had focused on me. I had to watch them kissing all the time and it was not a pleasant experience. I had never seen her like this before, and to me she looked stupid – what I thought of as soft and soppy — when he was kissing her. So not only did I not like the new house, I was not sure that I liked my father. He had never met a small child before and he had no idea what to say to me. I certainly didn't know what to say to him.

Because they were so absorbed in each other I had to spend too much time in the kitchen with Ivy Luker. Although Ivy had been a cook all her life, she cooked very disgusting food. She also had a very loud voice. When the meals were ready she would stand at the bottom of the stairs, by the door that led to the dining room, and shout out, 'I'm tiking it in!' It is hard to believe she could have done this with Uncle Wilfred and his rich banking colleagues: presumably he had a gong. This habit of hers made my father laugh — he thought the very fact of having a cook was funny, and he called her filthy Luker, although not to her face. I was rather shocked by this until it was explained to me that it was a joke because lucre meant money. It soon became clear that actually he and my mother were rather frightened of Ivy Luker. They didn't like the food she cooked but they couldn't bring themselves to tell her so: all our meals seemed to consist of boiled cabbage and meat in greasy gravy. She was also rather unattractive to look at, tall

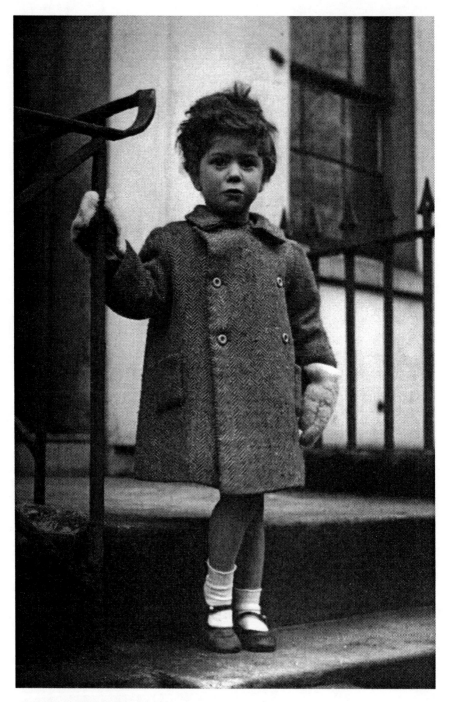

*Aged four, outside 32 Edwardes Square*

and fat with a faint but unmistakable black moustache. It would be years before they plucked up courage to ask her if she would like to retire.

My mother had had the whole house redecorated when she bought it, and, like everywhere she ever lived, it looked very pretty. The dining room downstairs, which had French windows leading into the garden, was painted terracotta red. When the neighbours came to visit they used to say it was very unusual. It was quite a dark room but in the evenings it was always lit with a large number of candles, some of which were held in the hands of rather battered gilded wooden cupids. On the ground floor at the front was the sitting room, where my mother worked — it had long velvet curtains and grey and white striped wallpaper on the walls. My father's study was at the back, looking out over the garden. He had a big desk piled high with papers, and a white pottery bowl where he kept his pipes — he had so many pipes that I couldn't count them. Best of all he had a theatre made of red meccano, with little string pulleys and handles to turn. This model theatre was one of the things that brought me and my father closer together: it was a toy, after all, even though he used it for his work, and he was wise enough to see that I must be allowed to play with it sometimes. I loved it when I was allowed to turn the tiny handles and watch various bits and pieces go up and down to what I learned to call the flies.

My parents' bedroom was upstairs. It was huge, with a sort of platform at one end with their big bed on it, and two large windows looking out over the square. At the back of the house was the bathroom, which had a grapevine growing outside the window: in the summer you could lean out and pick tiny black grapes, which popped in your mouth and tasted astonishingly sweet. Upstairs again was my bedroom, and very high up it seemed. When my first tooth got wobbly, my mother said I could make it come out easily. She tied a pillow to a bit of thread and tied the other end to my tooth, then she threw the pillow out of the window. I almost followed it out and had to be dragged back quickly. We didn't try that trick again.

There was a very odd episode in the first year of our living in Edwardes Square, to do with the room at the back of the house where my father had his study. He simply did not like being in that room, and every evening when he was supposed to be working he would pick up his books and papers and carry them into the sitting room where my mother was trying to draw. After a while they decided they really did need a room each, so she gave him the front room for a study and made her sitting room at the back. But then she found that she didn't like the back room and kept taking her drawing into the study in front where he was trying to work. So they decided to give the back room to me. I didn't like it either. It was big and rather dark and had red coconut matting on the floor, which scratched my feet when I got out of bed. Because I didn't like it in there I sometimes had a wee in a corner, on the coconut matting. It was also when I moved into that room that I started not being able to sleep. A baby-sitter told me to count up as high as I possibly could, but I got disheartened when I found I was up in the thousands and still awake. Sometimes I would get up and go to my parents' room and say 'I can't get to sleep', which must have been very irritating for them though they never said so. Then my mother would have to put me back in bed and tell me not to worry, just to rest. 'Rest is the next best thing to

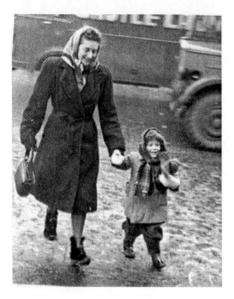

*Out shopping with Sophie*

sleep', she always said. After we left Edwardes Square my mother told me that they had decided that the back room must be haunted.

I was learning new words all the time. One word I thought was really funny was BELLY, which I had heard but didn't know the meaning of. Then one day my father came out of the bathroom without his clothes on. I was very surprised to see that there was something hanging down from under his stomach that swung about when he walked. I decided this must be a belly — it looked a bit like a bell, and perhaps some men could make theirs ring like a bell.

At this time in my life I nearly always wore dungarees. My hair was short and very curly, and I was rather thin because I was often not very well — I frequently had bad sore throats, which had been diagnosed as tonsillitis. People who met us in the street often thought I was a boy but I knew that I didn't have a boy's face. I sometimes heard people say I was pretty and I started to look in the mirror to see what that meant. I learned to make a face that I thought of as my pretty face, which needed quite an effort, as I had to think rather sad thoughts. I knew what it felt like but I didn't know what it looked like, because if I tried to look in the mirror while I was doing it, it didn't work.

I was learning fast, as people do when they are very small, and one thing I discovered quite soon was that my father was an actor. Not long after he came back from the war, he was in a play called *The Skin of our Teeth*, which I thought was an extremely funny name, as teeth did not have skin.

In September of that year I had my fourth birthday, and in the afternoon we went to see the play. I had never been in a theatre before and I found it wildly exciting to go in and sit on the scratchy red seats. Soon the lights went off and the curtain went swooshing up and behind it there was a great deal of bright light and a room with three walls, a door and a window. In the room, looking out of the window, was a very pretty lady with a feather duster. She said, 'Oh, oh, oh! Six o'clock and the master not home yet!' and a great deal more that I didn't understand. Soon a man came into the room, wrapped up in winter clothes. He had a moustache, but I knew who he was, and shouted out loudly, 'It's my Daddy!' People all round us laughed. I didn't understand the play very well but there was one bit I liked very much, which was when a dinosaur and a hairy mammoth were outside the house on the stage and were eventually allowed to come into the room. They kept saying, 'Cold, cold!' which for some reason made me laugh.

After the play we went out of the auditorium and into the stage door at the side, and found our way to my father's dressing-room. I was fascinated by everything in there: the table surrounded with bright light bulbs and the sticks of stuff that looked like crayons but were actually called make-up: it seemed that you smeared them on your face. I sniffed them and they smelled wonderful — I would always love that smell, and the feel of the white creamy stuff in a big jar, which was used to take the make-up off again. My father was going to do another performance later so he didn't take his make-up off, and I thought it looked very strange and orange on his face. I was beginning to like my father better now I had got to know him a bit: we were more relaxed with each other, which must have been a relief to my mother. Because it was my birthday there was a huge cake in the dressing room, and some of the other actors came in to have some cake and to sing happy birthday to me. One of them was the lady who had been on the stage at the beginning of the play, who was just as pretty off the stage as on it. Her name, I was told, was Vivien — Vivien Leigh.

At this time Vivien and her husband Larry Olivier were among

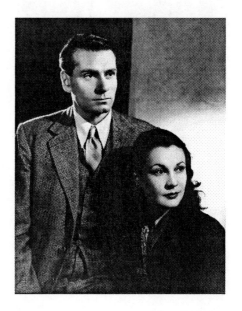

*Larry and Vivien*

my parents' closest friends. They had recently bought a big old house in the country, Notley Abbey, and one summer weekend we went there to stay. We had a big round bedroom in a tower, which was reached by climbing up a circular flight of stairs. This fascinated me as you could see how thick the stone walls were as you went up. All round the room were doors, one of which led to the bathroom. I thought I knew which was which and, making a dash for the bathroom, I opened the wrong door. There was a staircase right outside down which I started to fall. Luckily my mother was just behind and she grabbed me before I hurtled all the way down. Later, as we sat in the garden among the flowers, Larry turned to me rather flirtatiously and asked me a question: 'Who is your favourite film-star?'. Having recently learned what film-stars were I was glad to be able to show off my knowledge, but I only knew the name of one of them, so I said it: 'Stuart Granger'. Everyone laughed, including Larry, but I thought he seemed a little put out.

Larry and Vivien and my parents were always laughing. One day my mother told me about a dinner party they had all had together. An American actor, Danny Kaye, was there — I knew who he was because we had been to see him in a film called *The Secret Life of Walter Mitty*. When the pudding came, it was blancmange, and not very nice (perhaps Ivy Luker had made it). They had all tried to eat it, but suddenly Larry said, 'This pudding is disgusting'. Then he picked up a bit of it on his spoon and shot it across

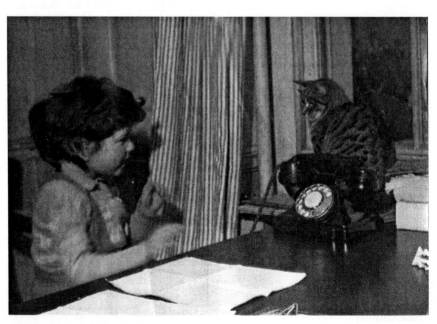

*Me and the cat in Edwardes Square*

the table at Danny Kaye. Danny Kaye picked up a bit on his spoon and chucked it back. Soon they were all throwing pudding at each other and screaming with laughter — crying with laughter, my mother said. I thought it was funny but I also thought grown-ups were very silly.

I had gradually got used to having a father. He was good fun when he was there, although he was always very busy and often out at work, even at the weekends. He tried to be rather stern with me sometimes, but I worked out quite quickly that he was really very soft-hearted and kind. One day when I would not do something my mother was asking me to do, he said quite mildly, 'If you won't do it, we shall have to make you do

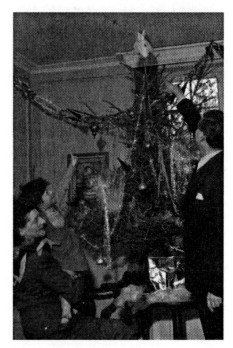

*Christmas in Edwardes Square*

it', and I said, quietly and confidently, in reply: 'Actually, you can't *make* me do anything!' When it was sunny we would sit outside in the garden and he would play a game with me, which he called The Grip of War. It was a simple game but I never got tired of it — he would imprison me by holding me tightly between his knees, and say, 'You are in the grip of war', and I would have to try to escape. He found out that it was easy to make me laugh, and he had a repertoire of jokes, which he used over and over again. Every time we had summer pudding for lunch, which was often because my mother made it so deliciously, he said, 'Summer pudding and summer not'. When we had to send our photos out to be developed, he always sang, 'Some day my prints will come'. Whenever we went past a shop in Kensington High Street called the Penguin Cleaners he said, 'I didn't know you had to send penguins to the cleaners'. Every time I heard these jokes I would giggle, even though I had heard them a million times before. When he came into breakfast with the newspapers – we had the Times and the Daily Mirror – he would roll them up and pretend to club me over the head with them. Once he dressed up as a lady in my mother's clothes, which did not fit him at all. I thought all this was very funny.

Edwardes Square was a good place to live, as it turned out. Our best friends, at number 33 right next door, were the Turners: Mark and Peggy and their children Catherine, two years older than me, and Christopher, whose birthday was just a week before mine. Next door on the other side was Bridget Cuthbert and her children Aiden, Binnie and Caroline. Their father was not there, and no one ever said what had happened to him. They seemed to be very rich, much richer than we were, anyway, and I was overwhelmingly impressed by the fact that they spent their holidays at a castle in Scotland. Caroline was the same age as Catherine Turner, and they both seemed huge to me. At first they ganged up on me a lot and played games I was not included in. Or if I was, it was not a very pleasant experience. They enjoyed making me play the game of pig-in-the middle, which in this case consisted of two big girls throwing the ball at each other over the head of a tiny girl who never ever managed to jump high enough to catch it. The worst thing they did, which upset me terribly, was that they somehow managed to stretch a piece of string across between their two houses at the back. It ran right across the back of our house, but their houses stuck out just a bit further than ours did and so it was too far out for me to reach. On the string they hung a basket into which they put secret messages. Then they jiggled the string and the basket went jerkily across from one house to the other: I had to watch it, but I could never see what was inside it. This made me feel really miserable and left out. My mother was sorry for me and tried to get me to make friends with Sally Oppenheim, who lived further up the square. She was about my age and everyone thought we ought to get on well but somehow we never did. When Cathy and I became really good friends, which we did quite soon, we started to leave Sally out of our games as she and Caroline had been used to do to me.

Until I was five I was often unwell and rather skinny. Once the doctors had found out that this was a result of tonsillitis, they decided to take my tonsils out. I had to go to the Great Ormond Street Hospital for Children. When I woke up after the operation my throat hurt a lot and all I could eat for a week was ice cream and jelly. After this I was not unwell any more and I gradually became rather round and plump. My mother called it puppy fat, which I didn't like at all.

It must have been around this time that we got to know a family who lived on the other side of Edwardes Square — the wrong side, Cathy and I thought. The father was an actor, like my father. His name was Griffith Jones, and he had a daughter called Jennifer, who had plaits and was about my age. Again, we were supposed to be friends, and again we did not really take to each other. One day I went there for tea and when I came back I was crying. I told my mother that Jennifer Jones had been horrid to me — she had said I was fat. My mother laughed and said, 'Well, that really is a case of the pot calling the kettle black'. I had never heard this expression and I had to ask her what it meant. Jennifer Jones ate a lot – once when she came to tea with us she ate nearly a whole loaf of bread – and she was at least as chubby as I was. We would have been surprised to learn that she would grow up to be a lovely (and thin) woman and a really fine actress.

I didn't think much of boys at this time. The one I knew best was Christopher Turner, who was horrible to me. He pulled my hair, hit me, and tipped my chair over backwards at tea-time. But on the wrong side of the square lived the only boy I admired — Bruce, who lived in the pub on the corner where Edwardes Square met Pembroke Square. He was a bit grubby-looking but he was good-natured and what was more he had one great point in his favour — he kept pet mice. They were white and he did not just keep them, he kept them hidden inside his clothes. They hid in his sleeves and in his pockets and up his jersey, and he scrabbled inside these places to get them out to show us. We never got tired of seeing the little lumps and bumps they made as they travelled on their journeys around his body. When I say we, by this time I mean Catherine Turner and me. Although she was two years older, we had started to like each other more and more.

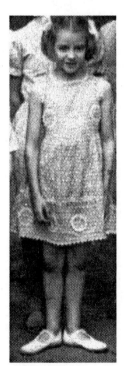

*Cathy aged about five*

She was clever and funny, much taller than I was and skinny, with a long, thoughtful face that I always thought was very beautiful. We played endlessly in the square, sometimes joining the strings of children glued to the railings on the side which overlooked the dark smelly lane, silently watching the men in raincoats who liked to show strange activities to anyone who cared to watch. We bought ice-cream from the corner shop, dull white squares wrapped in greaseproof paper which you had to unwrap and put between two flat wafers. In the winter we put on plays, at the Turners' or at our house. In one of them, I played a girl who was wearing some kind of Tyrolean costume, and I had to say: 'I have some nuts in this basket'. But when the time came to do the play, and all the adults were sitting down to watch us in the Turners' day nursery, I forgot to bring on my basket. I thought fast, and when my line came up I said, 'I have some nuts in the basket I have left by that tree over there', pointing off-stage as I did so. I was hugely praised for this improvisation: it was, everyone said, what a real actress would have done.

The Turners were the best friends my parents had in the square, though I was always aware that they were much grander and richer than we were. My father never stopped teasing my mother about her own grand and rich relatives, but they were nothing in comparison with the Turners, whose house was full of things which even I could see must have cost a lot of money. Ours on the other hand was full of things that were all very pretty but almost all slightly chipped and broken. None of us minded this in the least. In fact it was a source of pride and pleasure to my mother, and hence to me, that all the antiques were bought for 'almost nothing' in a wonderful, no longer existing, market in London, the Caledonian Road. The tarnished mirrors, the faded plates, the slightly rickety Victorian button-back chairs — 'Only five shillings!' — what a wonder. But Mark Turner — who would soon become Sir Mark because of something good he had done in the war — did not seem too grand for us, and in fact he and my father become quite good friends, chatting over the garden wall and sitting in each others' gardens drinking whiskeys while their wives drank gin and tonics. Peggy Turner was, above all else, a wife and mother. I did not know, and would not know for many years, that as well as being an astonishingly gifted artist, she was once an actress, and that she had sacrificed her career to do the right thing by her new husband, but this did, perhaps, explain the fact that she never seemed totally happy. She was pretty to look at, and quite kind and polite, but rather more cool than her expansive husband. She had a great many babies. As well as Cathy, to whom she was not, for some reason, very nice, and Christopher, whom she idolised, there was soon Baby Margaret, an adorable child who sat cooing in a pram outside the front door and was so pretty that she got photographed for a Cow and Gate baby-milk advertisement. When I was six, Peggy had two more babies, twins, Richard and Roger. Just before they were born she came to visit the school where I was, Miss Ironsides', as presumably she was thinking of sending some of the children there. When she came into the classroom where I was sitting, the entire class gasped — her stomach, in a floral smock, preceded her into the room by what seemed like several minutes. If anyone in that class of six-year-olds had any doubt about where babies came from, they had a powerful demonstration on that day.

It was lucky that, with so many babies, the Turners could afford a nanny. We didn't have a nanny, but we did have someone who was referred to as the 'mother's help'. She came from Ireland and her name was Josie Brosnan. She came to live with us when I was five, as by this time my mother had started working very hard — she designed three films and two plays in that one year. Josie was eighteen, and she missed Ireland very much. She taught me to say the name of the place where she lived, which was a white cottage in a village by the sea: Banogue, Inniscaul, County Kerry, Eire. She sang songs about Ireland and I learned to sing them too:

*If you ever go across the sea to Ireland,*
*Then maybe at the closing of your day,*
*You will sit and watch the moon rise over Glodagh*
*And see the sun go down on Galway Bay.*

Josie was well qualified to be a mother's help because she had nine brothers and sisters and had helped her own mother to look after them. She made my breakfast, took me to school, picked me up, and gave me my tea. My mother was usually home in time to put me to bed, where I went at half past six with a cup of cocoa and a piece of bread and butter, and had a story read to me. Josie had a sister, Bridie, who sometimes came to visit and later would spend a short time cooking for the Turners. But she was short and fair, not like Josie who had lots of black hair and thick creamy-white skin and the whitest teeth anyone ever saw, which, unfortunately, were full of holes, so she spent a lot of time at the dentist. Once a week she and Bridie used to go out dancing, to a place in Hammersmith that I thought was called the Garione but was really called the Garry Owen. This was the best bit of Josie's week. On those evenings she dressed up and this became the high point of my week too. She saved up her wages and every few weeks she used to go to Pontings, a shop in Kensington High Street, where she bought her dresses to wear to the Garry Owen. Then before she went out I would go into her room and watch her getting dressed. The dresses were always made from a shiny material which she told me was shot taffeta, and which changed colour as you moved in it: her favourite colours were red and green, which she said were Irish colours. The dresses had tight bodices and little belts, but the most exciting thing about them was the skirts, which were enormous — sometimes they were made from two whole circles sewn together. Then Josie could pick up the hem edges at either side and lift her arms over her head, and there she would stand, completely surrounded by sparkling, shimmering colour, just like the wings of an angel. Below the skirt were her legs, in stockings with seams (I was always useful here as I could check if they were straight) and shoes with very high heels and little straps round the ankles. On her mouth she would put the reddest of red lipstick, and I thought she looked very beautiful.

At first when Josie took me to school it was to my very first school, which was Kensington High School. I started going there when I was five, and it was not a happy experience. The lessons were alright, but the bad thing was what happened with the lunches. It all started one day quite soon after the beginning of the term when I had a plate of mashed potato put down in front of me. It was grey and watery and tasted very nasty so that I did not want to eat it — it had been made out of something that came in a packet, which was called Pom. You were supposed to mix it with milk and margarine but this had been mixed with just water. Because it tasted so bad I started mixing salt with it and soon I had mixed in so much salt in that I could not have eaten it even if I had wanted to. But then I found out that if I didn't eat it I would be in trouble. A teacher came along and told me I must finish it. I said I couldn't. She said I had to. I was frightened by now but I still said I couldn't. She said that if I didn't, she would have to take me to see Miss Baker, the headmistress. I was crying now but after putting half a forkful in my mouth I still said I couldn't eat the potato. The teacher picked up the plate, dragged me to my feet, and marched me to Miss Baker's room with her hand firmly on my shoulder. Miss Baker was sitting behind her big desk. She was short and fat and had an ugly, cross face with a nose that turned up and reminded me of a pig. Miss Baker said would I please eat the potato. I was crying uncontrollably by now but I said that I couldn't.

Next to Miss Baker's room was another room which was smaller and had bookshelves on all the walls. There was a chair in there. She told me to take the plate of mashed potato and sit on the chair. Then she said,

*You have to eat it. You will stay in that room until you have eaten it. If you do not eat it, you will not be allowed to go home. You will not be allowed to see your mother again until you have eaten that potato.*

I sat in the room all afternoon with the plate on my knee. I cried and cried but I couldn't even put a mouthful of the potato in my mouth. When the bell went for going home time, someone came and let me out, but I didn't tell my mother what had happened because I felt that I had been bad and I was worried that she would be cross.

Next day at lunchtime, when I was going to the dining room with the other girls, a teacher stopped me. I had been a naughty disobedient girl, she said, and I was not going to be allowed to have my lunch with the other children. I had to sit by myself as a punishment. So every day from then on I had to go and fetch my lunch, and sit on a chair in the library all through lunchtime, with no one to see and no one to talk to. This made me feel very miserable — I hated the school and I hated Miss Baker. But I still didn't tell my mother what was happening. All I did was cry a great deal, especially when it was time to go to school, which made my mother very worried.

At Christmas we were going down to Essex to stay with our friends the Collingwoods. Just before we left, my mother had a call from Miss Fitzgerald, my class teacher, who wanted to see her. So she sent me and my father down to Essex while she met with the teacher. A few days later, we were in the Big Room, decorating the huge Christmas tree, when she arrived from London. She came up to me straight away and put her arms round me and hugged and hugged me. Then she said, 'You will never, never have to go to that school ever again'. She looked as if she was going to cry. So after that one term I changed schools and went to Miss Ironsides', where I would be very happy for many years.

One really good thing happened to do with Kensington High School. While I was there, I made up a poem about Miss Baker. It was an act of revenge for the way she had treated me, and I taught it to my friends in the playground. It went like this:

*Miss Baker's deaf and dumb and blind,*
*I'd like to smack her fat behind.*

I found this poem very satisfying, and I chanted it to myself when things were bad. Many years later, long after I had left the school, I met another girl who was a pupil there.

*Do you still have a headmistress called Miss Baker?*
*Yes, we do.*
*Do you like her?*
*Not at all, but we have a good poem we say about her in the playground.*
*What is it?*
*Miss Baker's deaf and dumb and blind,*
*I'd like to smack her fat behind.*

It is impossible to express the pleasure I felt at hearing this.

# 3

Of the many things I learned from reading my father's letters to my mother, written throughout the course of their long relationship, one was the fact that the war helped my father to grow up. His letters from the 1930s, although witty and lively, show him as rather immature and very unsure of himself. Once he joined the army, his health improved beyond measure, as did his physical fitness, and he lost several stones in weight as a result of the regime. As an officer, with increasing amounts of responsibility, he acquitted himself admirably, even to the extent of getting twice mentioned in despatches by a hated commanding officer. His letters showed a huge increase in self-esteem. Gone were the self-pitying complaints about his attacks of ill-health, his bids for sympathy, his rather childish jealousies and his silly jokes. Instead of leaning on my mother for support, as he seems to have done somewhat throughout the thirties, he offered himself as a prop to lean on. There is not, in a single letter, any trace of irritation, of impatience – nothing, in fact, except unequivocal love. It is sometimes easier to love someone unequivocally when they are three thousand miles away, but the depth of feeling, the closeness, the passion, expressed in these letters seems to me to be unmistakable.

The other thing the war did was to give him a chance to think: to think about the theatre and his future in it. He had struggled in his early acting career, but by the end of the thirties his work was gaining respect and he had started to direct, with some success, and he had also participated in running a theatre school, the London Theatre Studio. His old friend and colleague Glen Byam Shaw, with whom he was in close communication throughout the war, was urging a partnership of some sort when they both returned home, but George had other plans. Essentially, much as he loved Glen as a dear friend, he felt that his work and his ideas were old-fashioned. The person with whom he wanted to work was the man he referred to as his '*maître*', the distinguished French director Michel Saint Denis. He felt that his long period of apprenticeship had just about come to an end by the last years of the thirties, and that he was now ready for a collaboration. But he wanted, too, a new kind of theatre, aimed at a new, extended audience. Like many people he had been brought for the first time into contact with a far wider range and diversity of the population than he had ever met before: 'these are the carpenters, the stage-hands, the people we never spoke to or considered'. It was to these people, ordinary people living ordinary lives, that he now wanted to bring the theatre. In a very real sense, the experience of war crystallised the ideas which would lie at the basis of the whole of the rest of his working life. In the event, soon after his return to England, George ended up working with both Glen and Michel. The three of them were offered the opportunity of running a theatre school and a theatre company under the auspices of the Old Vic Theatre: the Old Vic Theatre School and the Young Vic Company.

My own experience of life at this time was happy. My new school, Miss Ironsides', was a good school, warm and supportive. Catherine was an increasingly good friend to me. Admittedly my parents were always working, but my mother was wonderfully loving, good, and generous with her time and her affection. Since I was settled at school now, she managed to be there for me a good deal when I was at home. She worked at home a lot anyway, her drawing-book balanced on her knee, her little glass of paint-water within easy reach, her cigarette burning away in an ashtray. Her drawings were witty and delicate, and she liked to paint them very lightly and accurately. To do this she needed a fine point on her brush, and she would get one by popping it into her mouth and bringing it out tidy and sharp, though she used to laugh about the fact that she was probably doing herself no good by swallowing so much paint. Sometimes I was allowed to go to her work with her, to sit through rehearsals, to help her snip fabric samples in one shop and buy hat trimmings in another. I particularly enjoyed helping the wardrobe people by crawling under the big cutting tables and picking up pins on a huge magnet while the actors were having their fittings.

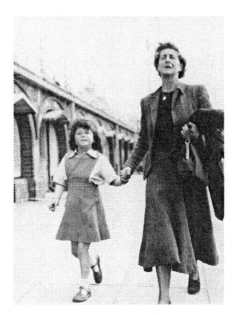

*Out for the day in Brighton*

We would sometimes go to my father's work, too. I was taken to see every play that was put on either at the Vic school or at the theatre itself. I saw *The King Stag*, *The Black Arrow*, which terrified me because it had a hooded leper with a bell in it, which would give me dreadful nightmares; *The Shoemakers'*

*Holiday*; and my favourite of all, *The Snow Queen*. This I took to be real magic, with ice palaces and talking ravens and people who were changed and lost and found. Another play which was magical in a different way was *A Midsummer Night's Dream*. There were fairies in this play but they were not pretty little things with wings, all in white, like the kind of fairies you saw in books — these fairies, designed by my aunt Percy, were like strange insects and birds, and they glowed in the dark because their costumes had been painted with luminous paint.

It was while this play was being rehearsed that I had my first taste of what it was like to be on the stage. It was during a lighting rehearsal. My father loved lighting — it was his real joy. At home he had wonderful little books full of

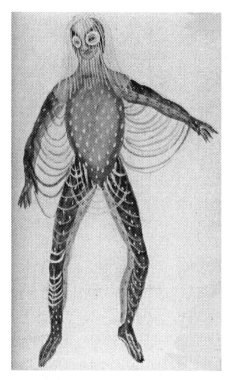

*Percy's design for Cobweb in* A Midsummer Night's Dream

things called lighting gels — small transparent squares of all the colours imaginable, all joined together at one corner so you could slide one out and hold it up in front of the lamp to see what the light looked like when it shone through it. I used to play with these for hours. But really they were for work, and my father used them to decide what colour the lights should be on the actors in the plays. Then he would sit for a whole day or more in the dark theatre with the set on the stage and call out to the people in the lighting box: 'O.P. spot — bring it up a bit — take prompt side spot down a bit' and so on endlessly. I really enjoyed this, watching the stage change colour and shape as the different lights came and went. So, aged about five, I was sitting quietly in the stalls when it came to the scene where Titania was going to sleep on her bank, before Puck put the flower juice in her eyes.

Someone needed to be on the bank so my father could light it properly but there was no-one about. Looking round, he saw me and said, 'Go and lie on the bank and pretend to be Titania going to sleep so I can get the lighting right'. So up the steps onto the stage I went, and I lay there, pretending to be a beautiful lady. But I heard some people laughing — not unkindly — and it made me feel a bit strange. Afterwards we were having tea in the canteen and one of the actresses came up and said that she had always thought I was a bit of a tomboy but that today I was a real girl. This did not make me feel all that much better. Perhaps, I thought, this acting was not as easy as it looked, but this didn't stop me wanting to do it, and do it better so people would not laugh at me.

Despite his wartime reservations, George was happy to be working in collaboration with Glen Byam Shaw as well as with Michel Saint-Denis. Glen was my godfather, and he was a lovely man, kind and twinkly — he limped a bit because of an injury to his leg in the war. Michel was less approachable. He and his beautiful wife Suria Magito, who had black hair with an amazing white stripe in it and wore lots of beautiful rings on her hands, lived just round the corner from Edwardes Square, in Earls' Terrace. So Michel was often in our house, and he and my father would sit together, both smoking their pipes and looking rather too big for the little Victorian chairs in the sitting room. They spoke French, because Michel was French and George loved to speak it. He loved it so much that he often spoke it at home even when Michel was not there, and he spoke it so well that, as I would discover a few years later, when in France he was taken for a Frenchman. Sometimes we had to speak nothing but French at meal times, and when I started to learn the language at school it was astonishingly easy for me. I was also allowed to have a little bit of red wine in my water at dinner time, like a French child.

My parents did love France very much. In fact that was one of the few blots on my landscape in one sense, since they wanted to go there for holidays and they did not want to take me, not when I was very little, anyway. They needed time by themselves. This was understandable from their point of view but unfortunately I did not see it that way. My mother's absences were unbearably painful for me. Even when she went out at night I was devastated, and quite capable of spending several hours in tears on the stairs, inconsolable until she reappeared. So when she went away for a week or more, life was simply agony. The first time it happened I was only four and the person who was left to look after me was my aunt Percy, who had just come back from America. I didn't have a problem with Percy as an aunt, in fact I was very glad to have her as I was a bit short of relatives. But she was no substitute for my mother, who had gone with my father to Michel's house in the South of France. I cried and cried and cried. One day, sitting in the bath, I had a momentary respite when I thought I hear my mother's voice outside the door, but it turned out to be Percy, whose voice sounded exactly the same, so this only made things worse. Percy was at her wits' end — she had no children of her own and I was the first small child she had ever had anything to do with. I lay in bed weeping and refused to get up. Then she had an idea. She telephoned to her friends the Guinesses, who had a boy named Matthew who was six, two years older than me. Could they bring him round to cheer me up? So up the stairs to my nursery came Alec, Merula, and Matthew, and there in front of them was this tiny creature, weak from grief, prostrated on the bed. Matthew looked solemnly at me for some time, obviously thinking what to do. Then he started to dance. There was no music, but he made the music in his head. He danced slowly at first, in a stately sort of way, but as he went on he got more lively and soon he was leaping about the room in a wonderful and astonishing way. I forgot to cry and very soon I started to laugh — the first time I had laughed since my mother's grim departure. So Percy's idea was a success.

I was a little older than this when I had a rather peculiar experience with a laundry-van driver. He was not our own laundry-man, the one who worked for the Brook Green Laundry and came every week with a hamper of beautifully clean clothes in exchange for our dirty ones, but he had the same kind of van. I was in the street, outside 32 Edwardes Square, when he drove by. He stopped just beside me, leaned out and asked if I would like to go for a little drive. He had a nice smile so I said yes, I would like that very much. So he helped me up into the passenger seat and drove off. He had a rather red face, and short hair, and small eyes. He drove slowly round the streets nearby, just round the square and into Pembroke Square next door. And as he drove he said, 'There's no door on your side, and I don't want you to fall out. So why don't you hold on to this?'. He took my hand and put it in his lap. His trousers were undone and there was something big and hard and red sticking out of them. So I held on tight and we drove around like that for a while. Then I said, 'I think I'd like to go home now'. He drove back to our side of the square and let me get out of the van. I said good-bye politely and went into our house. My mother asked where I had been, so I told her. She went very very pale and her eyes looked very frightened and very angry at the same time. She asked me if I could remember what the van was like and I could, not just the colour but also the name on the side. She went into the next room and made some phone calls. I couldn't hear what she was saying but I heard her voice, sounding agitated but firm, through the door. Then she came back and hugged me a lot and told me that man would not be working for that laundry any more. Then she told me I must never again go anywhere with anyone I didn't know, and I said I wouldn't. What happened on that day would always stay with me very vividly. Although I did not know what was happening, or even what this thing was that I was being asked to hold on to, I could tell that this was not what little children were usually asked to do. I thought to myself that the man was not bad or horrible, he was a bit sad, a bit like a child himself. He was quite kind, too, taking me back home when I asked him to. I was quite surprised, really, that my mother was so upset.

By the time we had been in Edwardes Square for a year or so I was used to living in London. I still loved the country, though, and luckily we managed to spend a lot of time there. This was because we had some really good friends who lived in Essex. They were the Collingwoods, the mother Kate and the daughter Teresa, who was one year older then me. Also living with them was Kate's mother, who we called Granny Edwards. As I did not have a granny, or at least not one who was any use, Granny Edwards kindly offered to be my granny too. Kate had been a student of my father's before the war, and she had got married to a man who had taught her at Oxford University. He was much older than she was and he was a very famous writer — his name was R.G. Collingwood. He had had another wife before Kate, and so Teresa had a brother who was older than her mother. R.G. had died, sadly, before Teresa was born, and Kate had moved out to the country, to The Clock House, near a village called Kelvedon in Essex. Kate and my parents got on really well, and we started to go to the Clock House every holidays. I liked it there more than I can say. It was a big old red-brick house with many rooms and it had a little clock tower perched on the top in the middle, which gave it its name. As soon as the school holidays started, my mother and I would get into our little car to drive down to Essex. The car was an Austin Seven, and really ancient. It was so small that my father, who was a big man, looked a bit ridiculous sitting inside it, and he and I had to get out every time we went up a hill and often also had to push it to make it get up to the top. But it got us about, even though there was no heater and the roof leaked, so that when it rained we had to wear our macs and even sometimes sit in the car with umbrellas over our heads and hot water bottles on our knees. We were often frozen to the marrow when we arrived at the Clock House, but Kate knew this and she used to have a

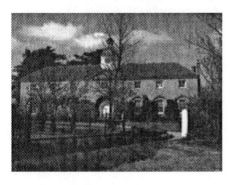

*The Clock House*

big pot of soup ready on the stove, a delicious kind of soup that she made out of potatoes and onions and milk with little green bits of herbs floating in it.

You never seemed to be bored at the Clock House. Outside at the back there was a courtyard surrounded by buildings — stables down one side and opposite the house a place called the granary, where the wheat used to be stored and ground, and which still smelled sweet and dusty, even though it had been empty for years. On the other side of the courtyard from the stables were big flower-beds, and a mulberry tree which dropped its great messy fruit on you if you sat under it in the summer. Over the other side of the wall was the chicken run — the chickens got to eat all our leftover food, cooked up in a pail, which I thought smelled surprisingly nice as it steamed away. Then, behind the granary, there was a big wild garden, full of bushes and shrubs, before you got to the iron fence that went along the edge of the back lane. Teresa and I used to play red indians out in the back of the garden, wearing little loin-cloths made from strips of torn-up sheet. One went round your waist and the other tucked over it at the front and back like a little apron. Teresa looked good in hers because she was thin and wiry, but I was beginning to get a bit chubby and felt rather self-conscious. We had bows and arrows, and we practised archery by shooting into a straw target fixed to the granary door. Teresa was better than me at this, but then she was better at everything. This may have been because I was younger: Teresa made no secret of the fact that she thought I was a baby.

It was out in this wonderful magical back garden that I got hold of the idea that you couldn't pray to God properly with your clothes on. I was keen on God for some reason – I liked my mother to say prayers with me at night, though we had never been to church. I decided, at the Clock House, that you had to be naked or God would not be able to see you as you really were. I built little altars and knelt down in front of them without my clothes. Teresa told me that a good way of testing your religion was to run naked through a clump of nettles. If God was really on your side He would make sure you didn't get too badly hurt. I really wanted to do this but I was too much of a coward.

All this happened in the summer, but even in the winter the Clock House was a wonderful place to be. There were huge roaring fires in all the rooms, and we played hide and seek in the day and card-games in the evenings – racing demon was a favourite, and reduced everyone to screaming hysteria. At bedtime Kate read us stories by the fire before we went up to bed. Her choice of stories was often a bit worrying for me. One had two characters in it called Death and the Devil which was scary enough, and another was *The Pilgrim's Progress*. I found this absolutely terrifying, and had nightmares about growing a big burden on my back and having to go to awful places like the Slough of Despond. Teresa made us try it, tying big bags on our backs and making me trek for hours through the bushes at the end of the garden.

The best time of all at the Clock House was Christmas time. We had all the usual things: a goose, generally, with everything imaginable that was good to go with it, and a huge Christmas tree that we had to dress up on Christmas Eve. It stood in the room that was known as the Big Room, and you needed a ladder to put the angel on the top. One Christmas day the weather was so warm that everyone sat outside on the steps in shirtsleeves and the grown-ups drank white wine in the sun. Teresa and I always had so many presents that instead of stockings we had pillow-cases. We had to have identical presents or there was trouble, and Kate was keen on educating Teresa so a lot of the presents were practical things. My mother would buy them from an art and craft shop called Dryads. We got lino-cutting sets, scraper-board, and one year even little looms for weaving. But one thing I could have and Teresa couldn't was comics. I was addicted to comics and I got a great many of them. There was the *Eagle*, with Dan Dare and the Mikon, and *Girl*, and *School Friend, Dandy, Beano*, and *Radio Fun*, which was a bit mystifying as we never listened to the radio so I couldn't make much sense of the characters in the cartoon strips. I think the reason I was allowed to have so many comics was that my father loved to read them too. He liked the *Dandy* and the *Beano* but best of all he liked *School Friend*. It had a serial story in it called The Silent Three at St Kitts which was his favourite. It was about three girls who wore hooded cloaks and went around doing good deeds. He read this avidly every week, and it made him laugh. He said they

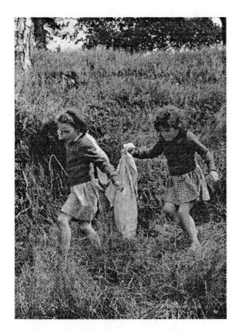

*Teresa and me at Aldeburgh*

looked like the Ku Klux Klan but I didn't know what this was. Kate thought comics were bad for you, and Teresa was only allowed to read proper books.

So when I was very small all our holidays were spent at the Clock House. When I got a bit older we became a bit more adventurous. One year Kate took me and Teresa to Aldeburgh in Suffolk, though as Sophie was working and did not come, I was rather sad and homesick. In the summer when I was seven, Kate and my mother took us to a cottage in Cornwall, in St Loy, on the south coast. This was one of the most magically secluded places imaginable. To get there you had to turn off a small country road and drive down a tiny, narrow lane, hardly big enough for the car and completely overhung with tree branches. At the very end you found a little cottage, very old and made of grey stone. This was the place we had rented. There was a small overgrown garden, full of ferns and fuschias, and on one side a path which led, in about five minutes, to a little rocky cove where no-one ever went except ourselves. It had a huge rock-pool where the water was warm and shallow, which I liked to try and float in as I could not yet swim. The whole area was full of huge hydrangea bushes, blue and pink, which I thought overwhelmingly beautiful.

The cottage and the cove were so safe and private that I was allowed to go down the path to the beach and back all by myself. One day I was happily walking along it when I was suddenly attacked by a swarm of bees. I started to scream, and Kate, who was luckily coming down the path just behind me, came running to see what was the matter. She began hitting at the bees to get them off me, and they started to attack her instead, even getting themselves tangled up in her great mane of grey and black hair. The two of us ran to the beach as fast as we could and dunked our heads in the rock pool until all the bees got drowned and floated off.

Close to the cottage was a sandy cove where we used to go sometimes, and at one side you could walk over the rocks at low tide to a second cove which I found terribly scary as there was an enormous wrecked ship marooned on a rock in the bay. The sight of this never ceased to frighten me. One day my mother and I had been exploring round there when the tide started coming in and we got into a bit of a panic about whether we would get back again. We sat on a rock for a while trying to figure out an escape route, and we made up a poem to cheer us up. The last verse went:

*Oh dear oh dear, I hope that this*
*Has been an awful dream*
*Because I know there'll be for tea*
*Cornish splits and cream!*

Luckily we did manage to get back and to have our Cornish splits, but Teresa had noticed how upset I had been, and that evening I saw her entry in the diary she was keeping religiously all holiday. She had written: 'I don't think Harriet would be very good in a crisis'. She was eight, a year older than me.

It was on this holiday that I had my first introduction to the facts of life. This came from Teresa. She told me one day that she knew how dogs mated and had babies, and asked me if I would like her to tell me. I said yes. She said, 'You know when men dogs have a pee?'. Yes, I did. 'Well, it goes hard and they push it up the lady dogs bottom and that's how the lady dog gets babies'. I found this quite astonishing, but I had imagined it wrong. I thought it was the pee that went hard – I could see it in my mind, like a twisted barley-sugar stick, dark yellow and thin and long. I could not begin to imagine how the dog could manoeuvre it into position. I never actually saw any of this going on but the idea of it stayed in my head for years. At least Teresa never suggested that people also did this – something to be thankful for — and I certainly never associated it with my experience with the laundry-man.

I read a lot of comics, but I read books too. I was proud of how well I could read. My mother had taught me when I was four, by showing me words in books and telling me what they said, and then getting me to find them again. It all seemed pretty effortless. When I first went to Miss Ironsides', aged five, they built me a special little bookcase in the class-room and filled it with books for me to read to myself while the other children were still struggling with their ABCs. I was happy at this school. It was in a street off the Gloucester Road, in a big white house with steps up to the front door and pillars. The two old ladies who ran the school were the Miss Ironsides, but like all the teachers at the school they got called by their first names, which were Rene and Nelly. Rene was the Headmistress. She was tall and straight-backed with white hair that rose high above her head before it got tucked into a little bun at the back. She was rather serious but she was kind and always fair. Nelly was small and soft and round, and looked as if she would like to give you a cuddle. Her face was round and wrinkly and reminded me of an old apple. Her hair was grey, and she tried to put it in a bun like Rene's but it remained wispy and untidy-looking.

Everyone was very kind at this school. My teacher was called Finny (Miss Finlayson, perhaps?) and she was the one who had arranged for me to have the special bookcase. Also I started having piano lessons, with a teacher who lived right at the school, in a little room on the staircase. Her name was Mrs Kelvin. We could call her Mrs K, but we were not allowed to call her by her first name although we knew it was Stella. She was from Germany, and had a strong accent. She seemed to me very old, and I was disturbed by the fact that her legs were very swollen. She kept her room extremely warm – there was a gas fire in there which was almost always on, and in front of it there was a crusty little bowl of water which slowly evaporated, so that Mrs K had to keep filling it up. It was there, she explained, to keep the air in the room from getting too dry.

I loved music and I was excited about learning the piano, but I was disappointed when I found out that all I was allowed to play were boring exercises. My mother went to see Mrs K and asked her if I could play some real music instead, so she let me play tunes by Bach and Mozart and I liked this much better. Mrs K said I was good at the piano but I should practise more. I never did, even though I went on having lessons until I was sixteen. Because I liked Mrs K so much, I persuaded my mother to let me buy her a present. We went to an antique shop and got her a little china figure of a naked cupid, which I thought she would like. But when we gave it to her, although I could see she was pleased, she told us that it was not the right thing to do: you were not, apparently, supposed to give presents to teachers. This made me feel ashamed and embarrassed.

I made some friends at this school. They were not as close to me as Cathy, but I got on with them fine. They were Carola Casson, who was slender and elegant, and whose father Hugh would design an opera for my father, *Troilus and Cressida*, and beautiful Georgina Howell, who loved horses passionately, and who would become a famous journalist. I learned a lot and I enjoyed the lessons, especially English and history. Maths was always a bit of a mystery, but everything else seemed very easy to me, a bit too easy in some ways, and the teachers seemed to think I was very clever. One day one of them said to me, 'Oh, I suppose you will go to university'. But the idea filled me with horror. I didn't know much about such things, but thought it sounded terribly boring, and besides, I wanted to be an actress, so I could be Titania on her bank of flowers and not have people laugh at me.

One thing I learned, though not as part of the curriculum, was the

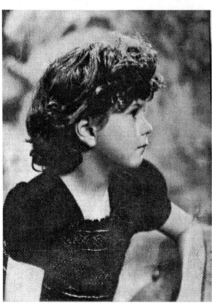

way people were supposed to behave about death. Two things taught me this. One was that the King died when we were at school and we heard about it while we were having lunch. Rene came in looking terribly solemn and said, 'Our King is dead'. We all stopped eating and looked sad. But I was very hungry and I wanted to know when it would be alright to take another mouthful. I looked around and guessed that everyone was thinking the same, but no-one liked to ask. The other thing that happened was that one of our teachers died very suddenly. She was quite old and her name was Miss Harvey. We were told in the

*Looking very pretty aged six*

morning when we got to school, and later in the morning we had a lesson about ancient Egypt. The teacher was explaining about the pharaohs and their dynasties, and she wrote the word on the board: DYNASTY. Someone laughed and said it looked like die nasty, and I said, 'I hope Miss Harvey didn't die nasty'. I was looking for a laugh, but I didn't get one. Instead the teacher looked sad and cross and told me I shouldn't say things like that.

I was about six when my parents decided I should have dancing lessons. Perhaps they had seen me doing my secret dances to the ballet-music records we had at home — *Coppelia, Les Sylphides, La Boutique Fantasque* — a little round person careering and twirling round the sitting room. I had seen all these ballets because my mother had a childhood friend, Joyce Boosey, whose family had a box at Covent Garden which we could use for nothing. I longed to be able to do ballet properly, and so I got sent for a short time to a place in Notting Hill called the Rambert School. Sometimes we were taught by the founder of the school, a tiny foreign lady whose name was Madame Rambert, who was very famous but to me seemed very frightening. She was always dressed in black, had her hair scraped back in a tight bun at the back, and she carried a stick which I thought she might at any time hit me with. She never seemed pleased with what anyone did, and made me feel even more chubby and clumsy than I already did. The Rambert School was too strict and serious for me, but the ballet lessons went on somewhere else all the time I was at school in London.

I got to dress up as a ballet dancer at my sixth birthday party, which was a very grand affair. It took place in a rented hall and there were a lot of children there, all in fancy dress. My ballet-dancer's tutu was made from black net, masses of it, all sticking out in what I thought was a very pretty way. Also very special on this day was my birthday cake, which was enormous, covered in chocolate icing with swirls and pink roses on top. It was so big that it got in the way in the little room where the party food was, so someone put it on to a chair. I was so excited that I ran around and bounced about, and I was so bouncy in the food room that I plonked myself backwards onto a chair, and then found to my horror that it was the chair where the cake had been put. I was absolutely devastated, and both the cake and my dress were ruined — the net tutu was absolutely the worst place for chocolate icing to end up.

I would never quite get over the desire to be a ballet dancer. Years later, when we moved to Hammersmith, I would watch the girls from the Royal Ballet School as they walked to Baron's Court station in little groups, their hair smoothly tucked into buns, their little feet turned out sideways. They all seem so slender and elegant, and they moved so beautifully, so much in control of their bodies. I craved for this but would never achieve it.

# 4

I suppose our first years in Edwardes Square were the most settled and peaceful years of my whole life. My parents were both working hard, as they would do all their lives, but I accepted this as normal, and they were certainly good value when they were around. I was, perhaps, a little sad at times that I was an only child. I think my mother had a pregnancy not long after my father's return from India, but this ended either in a miscarriage or a still birth – I have a dim memory of being told that I could have had a little sister, who was to be called Belinda, but that this was not now going to happen. Everyone else I knew seemed very well supplied with family of various kinds – Catherine, in addition to four siblings, had uncountable numbers of first cousins, uncles, aunts and grandparents. I only had Percy, a fine aunt but an unmarried one, and one extremely unsatisfactory grandparent, Granny Devine.

My grandmother, Ruth Eleanor Cassady, was born in Vancouver. When she married my grandfather she was twenty-three to his forty. She was a trained nurse, and as she was living in Liverpool when she was married, I suppose she must have had a job at one of the hospitals there. But the story I was always told was that my grandparents had met on holiday on the Isle of Wight. My grandfather had taken a break from the City to recover from a love affair with an actress, and Ruth evidently seemed to him a vision of freshness and prettiness: a picture of her at the period shows a lovely, dark-haired girl, elegant in her white muslin dress. According to my mother (my father never mentioned his mother to me) Ruth in her old age said that when she was a girl her father had said to her, 'You will not be getting married: you are not like the other girls'. What exactly this meant, if indeed it was true, is difficult to say. My mother took it to indicate that he saw seeds of her later mental instability.

My father was fond of telling a story that his mother had turned to his father after the wedding night and said 'You must never do that again', an anecdote which led John Osborne to refer to him as 'one-shot George'. Where George got this information is not clear, unless his mother made the claim in her sad decline. However, it unfortunately cannot be true, as my grandparents were married in early September 1909, over fourteen months before their baby was born. In any case, there seems little doubt that it

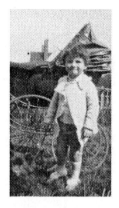

*Baby George*

was after George's birth that Ruth's mental condition became really unstable. Presumably this began as a case of post-natal depression, and it led initially to her leaving her husband and taking baby George to a retreat somewhere in the middle of the New Forest. Here she neglected him badly and subjected him to her fantasies about being pursued by the Prince of Wales, disguised as the milkman. I always think it is astonishing that my father survived this episode without suffering irreversible emotional damage, but I think he did survive it, although clearly it did leave its mark.

Rescued by his father, he and his mother were taken back to a quiet suburban existence in Hampstead Garden Suburb where he seems to have felt like a misfit on account of his short-sightedness, his ineptitude at games, and above all the obvious eccentricities of his mother, who was given to screaming at the neighbours as well as telling her son that his father was a bad man. George senior eventually moved out, and spent time with his son only at the house of family friends. It must have been a relief for my father to get away to his uncle Lex's rather seedy public school, Clayesmore, where he was virtually a permanent resident from his early teens to his adulthood, and in later life he saw as little of his mother as he possibly could. His wartime letters speak, in a tone of rather wistful tenderness, of occasional visits to her, but I never saw them together, as he used to disappear into his study when he knew she was about to visit, and Sophie was left to deal with her as kindly as possible. She had, by then, become a sad old lady in ragged overcoats (my mother said she still wore the clothes she had brought over from Canada for her trousseau, but this seems a bit unlikely and Miss Haversham-ish), with white wispy hair escaping below a dark blue beret. She was not what I thought of as a satisfactory Granny at all, though we called her Granny Devine. She seemed scarcely aware of me, and was probably longing to see the son who could not bear to be in her presence at all. By the time she died, in a nursing-home in Bayswater, she was unable to recognise anyone and on one memorable occasion took my mother (who was all of five foot two) for a Canadian Mountie come to take her back home, a development she seemed much to welcome.

I was eight when something very dramatic happened: the first thing that really disturbed our quiet and happy domestic life. Things started to go wrong at the Old Vic, where my father worked. Essentially it was a sort of battle between 'the Boys', my father George, my godfather Glen, and Michel, on one side, and on the other, the Old Vic Board of Governors.

Headed by Lord Esher and his second-in-command Llewellyn Rees, the Governors were trying to tell the Boys how to do their jobs, how to run the school and the theatre.

My parents, who always believed in keeping me in the picture, explained it to me in terms they thought I would understand. The Governors, they said, did not approve of the school because the students learned things like how to imitate animals and how to act in masks, which were nothing to do with what they considered to be real acting. And they were unhappy with the Young Vic too, because George's idea of taking plays to schools all over the country, so that children everywhere could have some experience of theatre, was not working. The schools he was writing to were just not interested and most of them did not even answer his letters. So Lord Esher and Llewellyn Rees told the Boys that they must change their plans and start putting on plays that would make money, but the Boys said no — this was not what the whole Old Vic Scheme was about. So then the Board got really angry. They found someone who would do things the way they wanted them to be done, and made him into a fourth director, to work alongside the Boys. His name was Hugh Hunt. But although Hugh Hunt and my father had been at university together, the Boys did not want to work this way. They believed that if they did, they would not be able to do the kind of work they were committed to. So they decided to resign, all three of them, and when they did, all the people who had been working with them and for them resigned also, and the school and the Young Vic stopped forever.

When the newspapers heard about this, there was a huge fuss. I found this quite amazing. Suddenly my father was at home all day, and he and my mother were tense and unhappy. Glen and Michel came round a great deal, and everyone smoked and drank wine and talked and talked. Then the phone started ringing, and my father kept answering it in a voice that got angrier and angrier, and slamming it down at the end of very short conversations, until at last it was taken off its hooks and left lying on the desk. It was the newspapers who were on the phone, and also they were at the door. Men (always men) in raincoats and hats, with notebooks in their hands, would be crowding up the steps and jostling each other in our tiny front garden, ringing the bell and knocking the knocker. At first my parents tried answering the door and saying things like 'No comment' and 'Nothing more to say', but the men kept trying. My mother came downstairs to the kitchen one day and said 'One of them just had the nerve to put his foot in the door', an expression I had never heard before and which fascinated me as it sounded very painful. The only way my father could go out was to climb over some of the garden walls at the back and escape through the house of a neighbour.

After a while the fuss died down and life got back to normal. Well, normal but different. Now George was not working for the Old Vic he had to find some way of earning some money. My mother was already working really hard, but what she earned was not enough for us to live on. So my father decided he would have to be what they called free lance. It was then that he started directing opera at Sadlers Wells and working each summer at the Shakespeare Memorial Theatre at Stratford. I loved going to the operas because I loved music, even though the singers were usually rather too fat for the beautiful costumes my mother designed for them.

It was around this time that I suddenly became properly aware for the first time of my mother's work. I had always known what she did and had even participated, in the sense of going to fittings and rehearsals, but I had never really noticed her drawings in any detail. But now, aged between eight and nine, I started looking at them properly and being amazed by how lovely they were. I loved the way she based them on paintings but managed to make them exactly right for the characters in the plays. Even the faces of the leading characters in her drawings looked just like the actors who would be playing the parts — she probably could have made a living as a portrait painter but she would never have thought she was talented enough. For *Hassan*, a very old-fashioned verse play by James Elroy Flecker which was not a success (in fact Percy described it as 'a complete and utter disaster'), she bought a series of postcards of exquisitely detailed Indian miniatures and spread them all over the table where she was drawing. And her designs were like another set of miniatures, with rich, bright colours and intricately patterned in painted gold. I remember little of the play itself, which was in heavy ponderous verse ('And at the closing of the day/Some to Mecca turn to pray/And I towards thy bed, Yasmin'!), though I do remember the very young actor Laurence Harvey who seemed to me very beautiful — a few years later, aged about twelve, I would fall desperately in love with him.

Later the same year she did the costumes for a production by Peter Brook of Jean Anouilh's *Colombe*. It was the first and only time she worked with Peter Brook and she found it very exciting: 'He strikes sparks off you', I remember her saying. For this production she used the paintings of Toulouse Lautrec, and her drawings themselves echoed the style of his paintings, even using his characteristic technique of shading one side of the picture behind the figure. By this time I had become very involved with what she was doing and used to sit beside her for hours watching the delicate paintings take shape.

A few months later she worked on her first opera, Tchaikovsky's *Eugene Onegin*, which my father directed at Sadler's Wells. Percy designed the sets, and Sophie was responsible for the very large numbers of costumes— one of the demands that opera makes is the fact the you have to dress not only

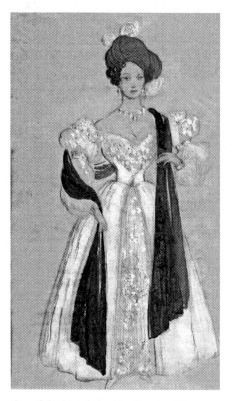

*One of Sophie's designs for* Eugene Onegin

the main protagonists but also the entire chorus. She really loved the challenge and was pleased with the result. The opera, based on a poem by Pushkin, was set in the 1830s, and she seems to have particularly liked the costumes of the period, managing to give all the ladies in the ball-scenes, for example, dresses which were different but which made a harmonious whole. Often, in this production as in others which made the same demands, she would do this by using variations on a colour theme — different shades of blues and browns in the *Onegin* ball, for instance. This same year she also did some beautiful costumes for a play that was thought to be too frightening for me to see: *The Innocents*, adapted from Henry James' *The Turn of the Screw*. I loved the designs, though, which were based on the paintings of Winterhalter, lush high Victorian, with ladies in enormous white muslin crinolines and huge hats.

So, by the time I was ten, I had seen a great many plays and operas in London. But this was the beginning of the Stratford years for both my parents, and it was Stratford that really made the biggest impression on my life.

On the very first of the Stratford years my father went down there on his own and directed *Volpone*, by Ben Jonson, which I was not taken to see. But the year after that, he was asked to do two plays, *King Lear* and *The Taming of the Shrew*, and Percy was going to be designing *Antony and Cleopatra* and *Richard III* for Glen, who was now running the theatre there. So my parents decided they would take a cottage for the season, and we could all go and live there. By this time I was nine, and they thought it would be alright for me to go to a local school for a term.

The cottage they took was in a tiny Gloucestershire village, Aston Subedge (pronounced subbidge, to rhyme with cabbage), which was twelve

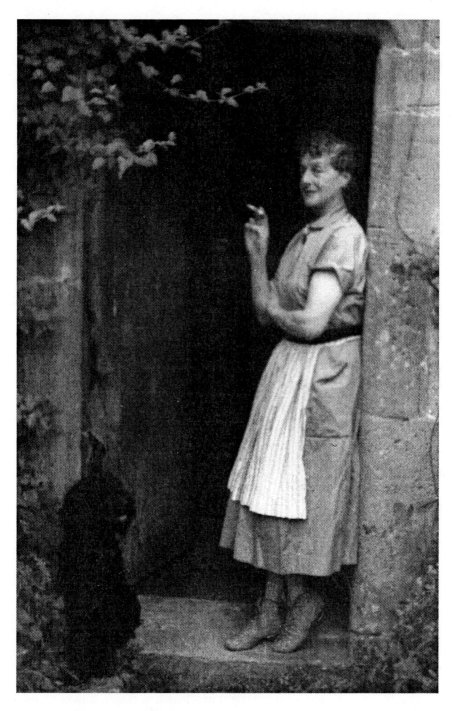

*Sophie with Alfred the dog at Aston Subedge*

miles away from Stratford. The nearest town was Chipping Camden, which was at the top of a very steep hill, and our village was the eastern (or Aston) village under the edge of the hill. The cottage belonged to some friends of my parents called the Bairds, and it was absolutely beautiful. It was about four hundred years old and was made of Cotswold stone, which glowed a sort of golden colour, and it had roses climbing all over it. Inside there were really low ceilings with oak beams, and stone floors. There was no electricity, and all the rooms had gas lamps on the wall which you had to go round and light when it got dark. My bedroom was tiny, and high up on the wall in one corner there was a little cupboard which proved to have a rope hanging from a beam inside. This always terrified me as I was sure someone had once hanged themselves off it. The cottage was on the very edge of the village, with fields and woods all around.

My mother was very busy that summer, designing a film. It was the story of the Australian opera singer Nellie Melba, and it was being very troublesome to her. The producer was an American, Sam Spiegel, and she described him to me as a very bullying sort of person. He disliked Sophie's costume designs as he thought they were not brightly coloured enough. One dress in particular, which she had designed in a very pale dove grey, he insisted on having re-made in bright purple. My mother protested, and when he asked her why, she said she was sorry to say so but the dress was now quite wrong for the period. At the time, she said, it would have been considered to be in bad taste. Sam Spiegel said, 'It's not a question of good taste or bad taste — it's my taste, and that goes!', a saying that became part of our family vocabulary from then on.

The amount of time Sophie was having to spend at the film studios meant that she was only able to be at the cottage at the weekends, and every Monday morning she had to get into the Austin Seven and drive up to London. On Friday afternoons I would sit in the front garden and watch the road winding down the hill until I saw her little black car come puttering down it. I missed her a great deal.

It was at the cottage in Aston Subedge that I first noticed how much Percy and Glen loved each other. I don't mean loved each other like a couple (although I suspect Percy may have been in love with him in the 1930s), but as really good friends. Glen was living in Stratford, but he used to come and visit us at the cottage a lot, and he and Percy would sit smoking together, sometimes talking, sometimes in a companionable silence. One day he got up to leave and looked out of the window at the torrential rain and said, 'It's absolutely *pouring* out of the sky!'. This doesn't sound particularly memorable, but I recall it with crystal clarity for some reason: this tall, thin, rather stooping figure at the window and the amusing, drawling voice.

Just before we came to Aston Subedge, Josie Brosnan had left us, though I never did find out why. Perhaps it was because she was finding it difficult to handle me as I got older. One day shortly before she left, she and I had a quarrel at breakfast, and I threw my fried egg at her and she threw hers back at me and we both burst into tears. Now there was someone else who had come to look after me, as an *au pair*. Her name was Christina af Bjorgsten, and she came from Gothenburg in Sweden. I loved her very much. She was tall and shapely, with beautiful curly red hair and a pretty, freckly face. She used to tell us that she was in England to find a husband, and was hoping for an English lord, though in the end she married a rather ordinary man – a commercial traveller, I think – and went to live in Scunthorpe. She tried to teach me a bit of Swedish: 'I Mai skol ya helsa po Christina i Goteborg', which meant 'In May I will visit Christina in Gothenburg', though I never did. We also thought it was very funny that 'Sit still' was the same in Swedish as in English.

So here we were in this idyllic cottage in this beautiful countryside and surely we must have been very happy. But there was one problem. I was going to school in Chipping Camden and it was not a success. I was simply not accepted there. My accent was wrong — too posh. My clothes were wrong — every time I wore a different dress there was an uproar of teasing and jeering, until I refused ever to wear any but one of two rather old and shabby ones. I knew too much — there were howls of disbelief and scorn when I injudiciously admitted to knowing French. The lessons, were in fact a waste of time for me because I knew it all already. The lavatories smelled dreadful. The school lunches were inedible, always composed of dried-up meat in gravy, lumpy potatoes and watery, tasteless vegetables. Pudding was always cake and custard, the custard tasting of caramel and very bright yellow, glutinous and runny at the same time. It was horrid but often the only part of the meal I could stomach. Luckily, unlike at Kensington High School, no-one minded or even noticed if I left parts of my lunch.

Of all the girls in my class, farmer's daughters all of them with carefully curled hair or plaits down their backs, only one, a very pretty girl with a pink and white complexion and admirable blond ringlets, seemed as if she might quite like me but mostly kept away for fear of what her friends might say. I did have one friend, and she was an outcast like me. Her name was Maureen and she lived in a dreadful little shack at the top of our hill with a huge family of equally scruffy brothers and sisters. She had only one dress, her shoes were in tatters, and her hair looked as if it had never been washed – all the other girls said she had nits, but I didn't think this was true. She had a kind brown face and though she was shy she was really sweet to me and we managed to make a sort of friendship. At least she was someone to say hello to and to go outside with at break. I have often wondered what happened to her.

As miserable as I was at the school, there was simply nothing to be done. So I had to stick it out, and I did. But luckily there were compensations. I fell completely in love with the countryside around Aston Subedge. Just behind the house was a bluebell wood, and part of the time we were there the bluebells were out. On warm days, of which there seemed to be many, I would go out and fling myself down among the flowers, just lying there with my eyes closed breathing in the smell which seemed to me to be unbelievably beautiful. I took care never to go to sleep, though, as my mother had once told me you must never go to sleep in a bluebell wood as the scent was so powerful you might never wake up again. On other days I would follow the course of the little stream that ran through the wood, scrambling through brambles and nettles in my wellington boots, until it disappeared into a hole in the hillside.

The place I loved the most was the big pine wood at the top of the huge sloping field behind the house. It was not as beautiful and varied as the bluebell wood, being just acres and acres of large dark pine-trees sitting on their soft bed of golden-brown needles. But it smelled rich and warm, and there was something so exciting and mysterious about it that I would go there all the time. It made me think about God. I had one particular place that I sought out, a little clearing right in the middle of the wood where the trees were suddenly in a circle with a little open space in the centre. To this place I would come, and I would scream. Not for any particular reason, though no doubt the tensions and unhappinesses of the school had something to do with it, but mainly because I just enjoyed the freedom of making as much noise as I possibly could. I told my father about it and he said he would like to see the place. So we went off across the steep, ridged field, into the depths of the wood, and I showed him where it was.

*And this is where you scream?*
*Yes.*
*Could I scream too?*
*Yes, why not.*

So he did, and I did — howling and screaming as loudly as we could into the great empty dark-green wood. I think we both enjoyed it.

George was a good friend to me at Aston Subedge. He was out a great deal, but when he was there we used to laugh a lot. It was here that he started an awful running joke that continued right into my teens. This was a forecast of my future life. I would, he said, be getting married to a bank clerk called

Clive, and we would live in Surbiton and have two children called Cecil and Cynthia. For some reason this made us both scream with horrified laughter, and I never seemed to get tired of having George perched on the end of my little bed telling me all about this dreadful suburban existence.

As well as going to school and screaming in the woods we went into Stratford quite often, and I got to see all the plays. Glen's two productions, *Antony and Cleopatra* and *Richard III* were designed entirely by Percy, presumably because my mother was busy with the film. The *Antony* was really impressive, and I think very much before its time in the sense that there was hardly any scenery, just a couple of pillars and some bits and pieces – a sail, an archway – that flew in to suggest the various locations. The play shifts constantly between Egypt and Rome, and Percy indicated this by simply changing the colour scheme – not just the actors' costumes but also the lighting, so that in Egypt the sky was blue or gold, and in Rome it was grey. My godmother Peggy played Cleopatra, a part which I think quite stretched her, and she did it superbly. *Richard III* I remember less well, though I do have a clear picture of Marius Goring as Richard, a terrifying figure with a chalk-white face and long, straggly reddish hair.

Perhaps my memory of the whole of this production is somewhat obscured by the fact that when I saw it (which I did many times) my attention became entirely focused on one single character, and not a particularly important one at that. This was Lord Hastings, and the reason I became so caught up with him was because of the actor who was playing the part. His name was Tony Britton and I fell deeply in love with him. Perhaps this may seem odd, as I was not yet eleven years old, but it was quite as real as any time I have fallen in love since. I knew him slightly, not well, but we used to meet him sometimes in the street, or at the theatre. I would sit for hours in the Green Room waiting in case he decided to come in for a cup of tea, and drag my mother past his dressing-room door in the hope that he might have left it open so we could at least say hello. One day we met him in a corridor and he and my mother had quite a long conversation. Afterwards she told me that I had gone completely white and had been trembling next to her all the time they had been talking. I am sure he never knew of my passion for him, but both my parents were only too well aware of it, as I talked about him endlessly, and knew all his lines in all his parts off by heart. Even now when I read them, I hear them in his voice, which to me was incredibly beautiful: 'Come, lead me to the block; bear him my head./They smile at me that shortly shall be dead'. Whenever we went to visit Peggy at her lovely big house by the river at Alveston I would make them drive slowly past the little white farmhouse where I knew he lodged, though it was set back too far from the road for me to see anything and I never even once saw him come out of the door. But he filled my mind and my heart, though quite what I imagined happening between us I am not sure – my knowledge of the facts of life at this stage was on the hazy side of non-existent and certainly what I did know seemed quite irrelevant to this grand passion. I think my dreams, day and night, were of some vaguely imagined merging into a union of body and soul, and that was as far as it went.

One good thing at least came of this obsession. Later in the summer my father's production of *The Taming of the Shrew* opened, and in it Tony Britton played the juvenile lead, a character called Lucentio. I think George did not think he was particularly good in the part (his talent, which turned out to be for comedy, would only appear rather later in his life), and in any case seemed to dislike him, for reasons which were not clear to me at the time although they became so later. So there he was on stage for a good long time, in a blond wig which did not particularly suit him, and I needed to commit to memory exactly what he said in his long speeches. To do this I needed a copy of the play, so after the first night I persuaded my father to give me his working copy. To say this changed my life would be an exaggeration, but it certainly had a profound effect.

The book he had been using to work from was an old Arden edition of the play, octavo size, in red hard covers, with Shakespeare's coat of arms embossed on the front. I read the play avidly, and I memorised Lucentio's speeches, which I can still say unhesitatingly today:

> *Tranio, since for the great desire I had*
> *To see fair Padua, nursery of arts,*
> *I am arriv'd for fruitful Lombardy,*
> *The pleasant garden of great Italy*
> *And by my father's love and leave, am arm'd*
> *With his good will and thy good company,*
> *My trusty servant, well approv'd in all.*
> *Here let us breathe* (here TB took a deep and stagey breath),
> *and haply institute*
> *A course of learning and ingenious studies…*

But possession of the Arden edition did for more than this for me. First of all it helped to understand fully what it was that my father had actually done to the play. Shakespeare's version starts with a trick played on an old tinker, Christopher Sly, who is transported, in a drunken sleep, to the nearby manor house and fooled into thinking he is the Lord himself, suffering from an illness which has made him forget who he is. As the Induction, as it is called, comes to an end, Sly is presented with some strolling players who are to act a play for him, which is the *Taming of the Shrew*. But then Sly and the Lord and all the other characters disappear, and the play simply goes on without them. What I learned from the Arden edition was that there was an older version of the play called *The Taming of a Shrew*, in which Sly and the attendants stayed on stage all the time, occasionally commenting on the action. This version George had incorporated into his production, so that the whole thing became what was called a play within a play, and on the stage it worked really well. So from this I gathered that a director could take liberties and did not have to stick slavishly to what the writer wrote, even if that writer was Shakespeare. But more than this I also discovered that it is not always easy or possible to find out what Shakespeare did write anyway. I read the introduction, I studied the notes, and I came away with a fair understanding of such things as good quartos, bad quartos (of which *The Taming of a Shrew* was perhaps an example), and folios. I knew who Heminge and Condell were. Also I realised that people do not always know exactly what Shakespeare meant even if they do discover what they think he said. These studies absorbed me more than I can say, and gave me the greatest imaginable pleasure. So I was in love with Tony Britton and with Shakespeare and with textual criticism. In fact all three were like a sort of magic circle which drew me in time after time and I never tired of seeing the play or of reading my battered Arden text.

At the end of this first Stratford summer, when my hated Chipping Camden term at last came to an end, we went on holiday to France. This was in fact my second French holiday, the first having been the year before when went to a villa my parents had rented in Roquebrune, Cap Martin, right on the Riviera. This had been my first trip abroad, and for me an amazing adventure.

We flew to France, my first flight, leaving Northolt airport in the middle of the night and getting to Nice early the next morning. The villa was lovely, very cool inside, surrounded by a rather dry little garden with plants growing in raised beds. An old lady looked after us there, cooking and cleaning. Her name was Madame Forestier and she spoke a language that was half French and half Italian – I think she may have been Italian. She took a great liking to me, and every time she saw me she would chuck me under the chin and say 'Che bella!'.

The beach was very close to the villa, just down a hill which had wide steps to walk up and down. On the way down you had to pass a gate which had the most wonderful deep purplish-blue flowers scrambling all over it. My mother told me the plant was called Morning Glory, which I thought was a very good name as it looked so glorious in the morning against the clear blue sky. On the beach I used to wear just a pair of swimming trunks,

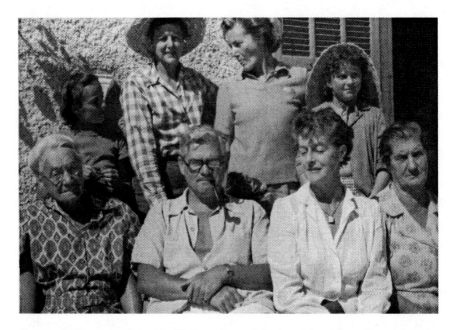

*Everyone looking rather discontented in Roquebrune. Behind are Teresa, Percy, Kate and me. In front, Granny Edwards, George, Sophie and Mme Forestier.*

all I had ever worn on any beach up to then. But for the first time I began to feel terribly self-conscious and aware of my rather chubby little body and of my breasts which, though they hadn't begun to grow yet, I felt should be covered up.

The beach was covered in stones, large flat ones that you could sit on quite comfortably. One evening when we got home my mother suddenly realised that she didn't have her cameo brooch, the one she always wore. She must have left it on the beach. My father said he would go and look for it, and she went with him to show him where we had been sitting. When they got to the place, he bent down and picked up one stone – and the brooch was underneath it. Another day my mother and I were out for a walk and we got a bit lost and couldn't find our villa. We met a lady on the road, and Sophie asked directions in her very best French. The lady answered, and they started having a conversation. After several minutes they both burst out laughing. The lady was English too but they had both thought the other was French.

Sometimes we would go to a different beach, just round the corner, which was busier and more lively. Here you could hire pedalos, something George loved to do. He would pedal himself out to sea and just sit bobbing on the waves and thinking, a rather large red-brown figure in the distance. We also liked it there because you could get chips, except that they were called *pommes frites* and much nicer (thinner and crispier) than English ones. Some days we would go and sit in a cafe in the town square and here it was that I learned to love *citron pressé*. You would sit under the plane trees in the square where old ladies in black sat in doorways and mangy cats you were not allowed to touch roamed the streets. The waiter would bring the lemons, cut in half, a lemon squeezer, a tall glass, a jug of water, some sugar, and a long spoon. Then you could make the *citron pressé* yourself. The sugar would take a long time to dissolve and you could watch it whirling around in the glass with little bits of lemon pulp. That was the good thing about French cafes – the bad thing was the loos which you had to avoid if possible because they were just a hole in the ground with two platforms for your feet and a cranky old chain overhead to make the water rush down the hole. They were never clean and always smelled very bad indeed.

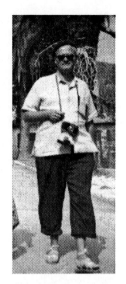

*George in French mode*

It was in Roquebrune that I first saw my father in his fully French mode. As he spoke French so perfectly no-one ever knew he was an Englishman and that made him very happy. In fact I think he would have been pleased if he had always been taken for a Frenchman. He always wore a beret – he had two of them, one an ordinary small one and one a large flat one known as a *beret basque*. And in truth he did look just like a Frenchman, with or without the beret, striding up the mountain side, his favourite form of relaxation: he would go for long long walks, off into the distant perfumed countryside among the wild thyme and the olive groves. Now I knew what he and my mother had been doing every year when they disappeared to France to stay with Michel or in some little hotel somewhere, leaving me ill and desperate with whoever was unlucky enough to be left to look after me. He loved the sun, too, and I remembered one holiday when I had been left behind, when he had written me a delightful letter illustrated with a series of pictures of himself gradually turning red, then red-brown, then dark brown. Now I was able to witness this process for myself. He enjoyed teaching me French phrases: '*Cher ami, tu sais, je veux des tomates farcies*', for example, which had to be said in a rather coyly flirtatious manner.

When I had been taken once, I was not left behind again. The second year — the Stratford year, the Tony Britton year — we went by car. When I heard we were going back to France I hoped it was Provence again as I had loved the smells and the colours and the sea. I was disappointed when

I found we were going to the Dordogne, even though my parents told me I would enjoy being by a huge river where I could swim, and in fact for some reason the holiday was not a huge success. I suspect that my father was already in a rather confused state, unsure about the future of his marriage, though this was never even hinted at. The first bit was most enjoyable. We drove to the south coast of England, and put the car onto a tiny plane which had a front which opened. The plane just hopped over the channel, from Lydd to Le Touquet. Then we set off to drive south. In the car were me, my mother and father, and Christina af Bjorgsten. I was very taken with the long straight French roads all lined with poplar trees, and the farmhouses set back in the fields, and the old men in dusty blue on bicycles with bags of tools or long loaves of bread. Sometimes, I was pleased to observe, they would get off their bicycles and have a pee by the side of the road.

Because I was in love with Tony Britton I couldn't stop talking about him and this drove my parents mad. One day I saw a white farm which looked very much like the one he lived in at Stratford and I said with rather self-conscious innocence, 'Oh, that farmhouse really reminds me of something', and my father said, 'I suppose it is Tony Britton's face'. This was the first of many times I would find out how hard it is not to talk endlessly about the person you are in love with and how much other people get irritated by it. You think they will not notice but they always do.

For some reason no-one seemed to be enjoying themselves as much as they should, or perhaps George was just afraid that they wouldn't. He kept asking us to reassure him that we were happy — we had to say loudly, in chorus, '*Nous sommes heureaux*'. But this holiday seemed not to be a particularly happy one. We were staying in a hotel in a village, Beynac, right on the banks of the Dordogne, and it was really beautiful place. You could swim in the river outside the hotel and the houses were reflected clearly in the still flat waters. The hotel was small and run by a widow and her daughter who looked after us really well and cooked delicious food. I expect George found it in the *Guide Michelin*, where he always sought out small family-run hotels with good food. One day Madame cooked us the speciality of the *maison*, a dish called *Lievre a la Royale*. This was a whole hare cooked in an amazing red wine sauce, and it was quite the richest food I had ever eaten. As I had rather a delicate stomach it made me ill and I had to spend the next day in bed. Madame was very sorry and concerned and kept coming to my room with pots of camomile tea. This was the first time I had ever tasted this drink and though it did me good and I recovered quickly I would never enjoy it very much in the future because it would always remind me of being ill in the Dordogne. And I would never eat *Lievre a la Royale* again.

On the way home we drove back through Limoges. My mother had looked forward to this because famous china was made there, but it turned out not to be a very nice place at all. This was the only time on holiday with my parents that we ever stayed in a big hotel in a large city. After two weeks in Beynac it seemed very busy and grey and noisy and full of cars. There were a great many soldiers in the city for some reason — they must have been on leave from a billet nearby. Some of them were black, and these were the very first black men Christina had ever seen — they did not have any in Gothenburg, apparently. She was absolutely terrified just at the sight of them, and kept saying '*les negres, les negres*' (I'm not sure why she said it in French, unless perhaps my father had been teasing her about them). She cowered down in the back seat while we were driving through the streets, and was very agitated all the time we were in Limoges. We had to stay in the hotel room in the evening as she was afraid to go out into the streets.

# 5

When we went home to England, it was not to Edwardes Square. My parents had decided to sell the house at the beginning of that year. This decision was all laid at George's door. He said the house was dark and claustrophobic, and he wanted somewhere big and light with huge windows. I suppose he was right about Edwardes Square – it did, after all, have the haunted bedroom – but the place we moved to was not really right for us either. It was at number 85 Addison Road, and it was a flat that was on two floors, the ground floor and the basement, which had a garden at the back. The house was huge, late Victorian, and covered with white stucco. The two front upstairs rooms were my bedroom, on one side of the front door, and a big studio living room on the other side which went right through to the back of the house and had a window which overlooked the garden. My parents' bedroom was behind mine, and downstairs were the kitchen and the dining room and Christina's bedroom.

It was at Addison Road that we first started to keep pets. We had two budgerigars in a cage hanging in the living room window, and the first winter we were there the weather was very cold. The birds seemed to be suffering so my father thought they should be given some brandy to warm them up. They sipped away at it, and then they got terribly drunk and reeled around their cage for a bit, then they both fell down stone dead on the floor. We also had a poodle called Alfred, whose pedigree was impeccable but who had come cheap because his tail had been chopped off too short when he was a puppy. We never had him shaved, so he was a wonderful, untidy bundle of black curls. George loved him and he loved George. They used to sit in the kitchen gazing into each other's eyes, and my father would say, 'Speak to me, Alfred, speak to me! I know you can!'. But Alfred never did.

We never seemed to warm to Addison Road. For one thing my father was evidently going through some kind of crisis, what would now be called a mid-life one, perhaps. Probably this had something to do with his frustration with his working life, as he had lost the Old Vic and had not yet found anything to do which fulfilled his desire to be more than just a director and actor. He was directing, a great deal, and he was acting too. He appeared in plays at Stratford and in the West End, in films, and in one memorable television play which was directed by someone he had just met, a young and eccentric director just down from Oxford called Tony Richardson.

This was an adaptation of a short story by Chekov, *Curtain Down*. George played an old actor who had a heart attack backstage and was slowly dying, in costume, throughout the play, although his fellow-actors believed he was simply drunk. As we did not have a television, we went to the Turners' to watch it. This was for me the most agonising experience – this man, sick and in pain, unable to get anyone to take him seriously, slowly slipping out of his life. And it was, though we had no idea of it at the time, a terrible prevision of what would happen to George himself some fourteen years later. But despite being as busy as usual, he was not satisfied. He was a planner, a campaigner, perhaps even a visionary and he needed a proper scope for all this. It was around this time that he started planning what was called the Court scheme with his new friend Tony Richardson, but initially his plans did not work out, which must have been difficult to take.

So I think perhaps this crisis influenced the way he suddenly took against Edwardes Square, and also the fact that he obviously wasn't very happy on the Dordogne holiday. Also, however, there seems to have been a more personal aspect to the whole thing: it seems to have been in Addison Road that my parents' marriage started to go wrong. This is only guesswork, as it was still many years before anything actually happened. But two things make me think this. One was the fact that my father started on his tremendous diet at Addison Road. The diet was a great success, and within a year he went from being a large fat man to being a tall slender and elegant one. He seemed to do this largely by eating Energen Rolls, which were a little like bread rolls but a good deal wispier. They looked as if they might be delicious but in fact they were disgusting, as they dissolved into nothing when you bit into them. I was also in need of losing weight, so I tried to join him on the Energen Rolls, but they were so horrid that I had to put a lot of butter and jam on them and then somehow they didn't seem to work.

The other thing that makes me think there was some kind of personal crisis going on which was connected with my parents' relationship was a book which suddenly appeared on the bookshelf called *A Modern Pattern for Marriage*. It was from this book that Catherine and I learned the facts of life. Certainly my mother was too shy to talk to me about such things though I know she wanted to. She did manage to tell me about something called the curse, and it was just as well that she did as soon afterwards I started having it. It was horrid and embarrassing, and I was the only one in my class to have it, or at least I thought I was, though nobody ever discussed anything so personal.

Catherine and I had managed to pick up a bit of information about what human beings do together in bed, though I suspect she was rather more knowledgeable than I was, probably because she was two years older.

But it was the *Modern Pattern for Marriage*, which must have been one of the most boring books imaginable, which gave us the details, albeit in a very dry form. It did this in one chapter, which we read and read until we knew it off by heart. This was the chapter that described what married people did in bed:

> *The man takes his position over her, his knees inside hers. With his right hand he guides his penis to the vaginal entrance, and makes his entry slowly and gently.*

This last phrase became a chant, which we would sing, quietly over and over again: 'he makes his entry slowly and gently'. It almost rhymed, which made it particularly appealing. I have never known if the book was put there for us or whether it was something my parents were using to help their own relationship. I rather hope that they hoped I would read it, because if not, they were letting me grow up in total ignorance of something which surely they must have realised was important for me to know.

Obviously my parents didn't need the chapter on sex because they knew how to do that. But presumably the other stuff in the book – the bits we found excruciatingly boring – must have been about how to sustain a relationship. If so, they clearly were not very effective. I'm afraid the truth may be that, fond though my father still clearly was of my mother, he simply had stopped finding her sexually attractive: the ten-year age-gap finally coming to matter.

It is only quite recently that I have come to know more of the details of my parents' early relationship. I have said that they were instantly attracted and that they started a love affair almost at once. But, reading George's letters from the summer of 1932, when the three girls were spending a summer holiday in Cornwall, it seems clear that he had fallen in love with the Motleys *en masse*.

He was stuck in London, playing a small part in a production at the Queen's Theatre, and with the help of his new friends was furnishing an unattractive bedsit he had taken in Litchfield Street. However he managed a flying visit to St Mawes and was obviously swept off his feet by them all over again:

> *was all the loveliest dream I have ever had — to be in a lovely place alone with lovely people. And to be free, and sail, and shout and laugh, all at once, without minding anything else — quite a time one cannot expect to last for more than a day. But I shall never forget it — even if I come to forget the Motleys — but I don't see how one can forget people who give one a little piece of mad heaven now and then.*

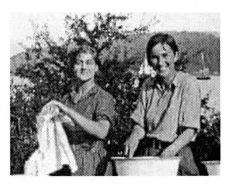

*Sophie and Liz at St Mawes, summer 1932*

These early letters are written to all three of them, though there are passages addressed just to my mother which are full of private references and deliberately tease Percy and Liz ('This will get the other girls guessing...I bet Percy is blushing now with sheer curiosity, and Liz is pretending she isn't interested'). He addresses them all with a mixture of risqué jokes, effusive declarations of undying love and sudden moments of painful self-doubt. The bits that are just for Sophie have an intimate tone which is at this stage teasing and sexy rather than tender, and which easily tips into insecurity ('Are there any men at St Mawes... — because I shall feel very jealous...Are there any men with whom you consort'). He alternates between schoolmasterly, scolding Liz for her terrible spelling ('dreadful not dreadfull...Isn't not Ise'nt'), and schoolboyish – even his suggestions for the planning of the sets for Gielgud's forthcoming production of *The Merchant of Venice* at the Old Vic are heavy with sexual innuendo. Advising them on the best use to make of the 'large phallic symbol which forms the centre of the of the stage, and which is more generally referred to as "the large pillar already at the Vic"', he says it is:

> *rather mediaeval, Norman, heavy, baronial, obscurantist, un-'gay Venice' and all that...I dare say it could be lightened up a bit by some skilful Motley brain work, but I don't somehow connect Venice with thick heavy round erections. I may be and probably am wrong*

And already he had started to make himself useful to them in a practical way by helping them with their accounts, something he would do for them for years, until his acting career really took off. Even here he cannot resist an appeal for love and sympathy. For their very first London production, André Charlot's production of the unmemorable comedy *Men About the House* he reported that they had made a net profit of £16, and one of £7 for the two Sunday performances of *Richard of Bordeaux* in June (the play opened for a run at the New in February of the following year). A total of £23, which, divided equally between the three Motleys, gave them £7-13/- each. But he adds, they owe: 'Debts to George for love rendered £7-10/- each. Net profit each = 3/- (Now buy yourselves new bathing costumes!)'.

By 1933 the Motleys seemed to be on an irreversible road to success. Their first tiny workshop in Duke's Lane, Kensington, proved to be too small and they moved to their celebrated studios in St Martin's Lane while they were working on Gielgud's *Richard of Bordeaux*. Once the workroom of the eighteenth-century furniture designer Thomas Chippendale, the studio, with its cobbled yard, became a centre where all the young actors, writers and directors would gather for tea and conversation. Alec Guiness, who met the Motleys in 1934, remembered the studio with gratitude and affection, as he wrote to me not long before he died:

> *Sophie and Percy were enchanting. Your mother's eyes would water with giggles very rapidly I remember — or if not always with giggles then from the cigarette smoke which always surrounded her....They were hugely generous and dispensed tea and cakes in their studio daily to impoverished actors like me who dropped in endlessly. But it wasn't just our greed — it was for the company of Sophie and Percy.*

My father soon moved in with them, and he and my mother became an accepted couple. There are still letters, written from distant places, tours with plays, or holidays. After a while the letters were just written to my mother – 'I love you most dearly, beloved' – and it is clear that he missed her terribly. Parted from her in September 1934, when he took a holiday in Paris, he wrote copious letters almost every day he was away. His first is dated 15.55/90 MPH/4,600 ft altitude/70° F — a testimony to George's excitement at being on his first flight. His letters swing from the jocular to the reflective — he thinks Paris 'gives more incentive to any kind of artistic outlook' because there is so much to see that is attractive and because he thinks the French have a more high developed critical faculty. He also feels less foreign: 'What a boon for a character actor: there are so many types that seem to be in my line here but in England so few'. One delightful letter is written during a meal, on a piece of torn-off paper tablecloth smeared with samples of what he is eating: '*oeufs au plat nature*, 3 Fr, looking good, *hein?*...here is the *Chateaubriand* and here the watercress. While I am on the subject you may as well have some of my *Vin Rouge*'.

As far as one can tell from the letters written through the 1930s, my parents' relationship was happy and intimate. George writes warmly and lovingly, and his early insecurity and jealousy largely to have disappeared. James Cairncross, who was an acting student at the London Theatre Studio, remembered with 'infinite joy' being taken back for an evening meal at the house in Islington where George lived with the Motleys: 'It was the first time I had ever dined by candle-light; and I remember George beaming round the table and saying, "I adore these evenings"'. This occasion, which must have been some time in 1938, sounds delightfully happy and domestic. But in early 1939 something happened which caused my parents to separate.

The facts are not easy to ascertain. I knew nothing of this episode until I read George's letters and discovered a small batch of them, four in all plus a telegram, dated from January to August 1939, which clearly indicated that they were no longer together. I was puzzled by these letters at first. My parents were evidently not seeing each other and my father was obviously tense, confused, and miserable. The first one is dated 31 January 1939:

*My darling —*
*Thank you for your letter: it helped a lot. It upsets my balance rather when I see you because it is so difficult to keep right when one is lonely and troubled. I would like to meet again soon — but not just for a little bit.*

He was lonely because, for the first time since 1932, he was living alone in an unpleasant overheated apartment, waiting to move into a flat which he was thinking of taking, in Mecklenburgh Square, Bloomsbury. Obviously missing Sophie dreadfully, he confided the details of his ill-health ('I had one of my liver attacks last night, but fortunately quite a mild one'), the fact that he was 'exhausted' and felt 'weak and disorganised'. In his third letter, written on 22 April, he suggested they 'try and meet normally for a while' as 'the situation' was becoming intolerable for both of them. But what situation? The fourth and final letter, dated 5 August and written from Saint Denis's house in the South of France, goes some way to revealing what I had begun to guess: George was involved with someone else. 'Annette was very kind….Annette left for Brittany'. His health was still bad ('I had one of

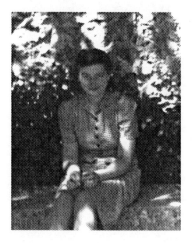 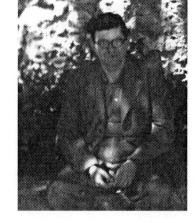

*Annette and George in the South of France*

my usual collapses'), but after a 'relaxing and not excessively happy' week he was feeling better in health, and:

*beginning to feel clearer and to know that I must never again get into the state I was in. Talk about a muddle…..As to a solution to my private life, I am at least clear that I have not got one.*

It seems evident, then, that George had got involved with Annette Scott – a design student at the London Theatre Studio – but had not been sure that he wanted to give up Sophie. Sophie, perhaps rather intelligently, had insisted he move out of the house and had indeed refused to see him until he made a decision. Really one cannot be entirely surprised at his falling for someone else: he had, after all, been with Sophie for seven years, since he was twenty-one, and some kind of restlessness was probably understandable under the circumstances. But what emerges from his letters is how deeply he was still dependent on Sophie, even if this was partly a kind of filial dependence, as his reiterated references to his illnesses suggest. The subtext seems partly to be that no-one apart from her could really understand his problems and his needs. Without Sophie's letters, which sadly no longer exist, it is difficult to know exactly how she handled all this: Percy, when pressed for information, remembered the incident but said that Sophie did not confide in her. One thing Sophie did do was to take holidays. She went to Ireland with Peggy Ashcroft in February and, so it seems from a couple of references in George's wartime letters, may have had a brief fling while she was there, and then she was in Nice in August.

Whatever the truth of all this, George's holiday in France seems to have sorted things out, and a week after his final letter he appears to have come to a conclusion. This at least is suggested by the telegram he sent to Sophie, who was still staying with her friends in Nice. Dated from Paris, 12 August, it simply says: 'Am staying Hotel des Saints Peres Rue des Saints Peres until Tuesday would like us to meet'. After this the letters stop, and my parents were married just over two months later, on 27 October 1939. Presumably plenty of rest and relaxation, and long talks with Michel and with Glen, who had joined them in France, finally helped him to decide what it was he really wanted, which turned out to be marriage and domesticity in his new flat at 35 Mecklenburgh Square. Quite why they decided to go for marriage after so many years of cohabitation is not recorded, but I would imagine it had something to do with the declaration of war with Germany in September 1939, an event which made many people think more seriously about the future.

Certainly George's wartime letters show that he missed my mother terribly, and my own memory of my parents as they were when I was small suggests that their relationship continued to be surprisingly (to me embarrassingly) passionate in the early years after his return. But his troubled state around the time of our move to Addison Road suggests that things had begun to change. Percy told me once that she thought that it was around this time that he started to fall in love with someone else. Whatever the truth may be, these Addison Road years certainly saw the beginning of my father's personality change, if that is not too strong a word.

We stayed at Addison Road for only about eighteen months. The flat was rented, and the money from Edwardes Square was waiting till my parents found another place to buy. And, when I was eleven, they came back from a day out and told me that we would be moving. They had found a house and had fallen completely in love with it. It was 9 Lower Mall, one

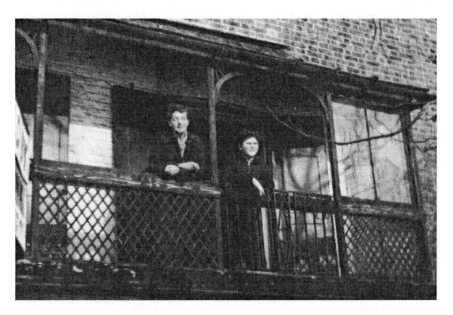

*With Sophie on the balcony of Lower Mall the day we moved in*

of three eighteenth-century houses with balconies right beside the river in Hammersmith. Soon after this I was taken to have a look at it. Built in 1714, reputedly for a mistress of George I who was being imported from Germany, the house had no road in front of it, just a towpath alongside the river. Our balcony was painted black, and you got out onto it through one of two sets of French windows in the first floor sitting room. This room was a very pretty shape, with walls with little scooping curves in them, and Sophie made it look lovely with regency striped wallpaper, Victorian furniture, little wall-mounted candelabras, and those battered gilt cupids above the windows. The hallway and the stairs were hung with prints of Impressionist paintings , mostly Toulouse Lautrec posters, but also Rouault's Clown, a painting I found terribly sad and disturbing.

It was at this house too that I first discovered that my mother could get just about any plant to grow. Lower Mall had a small garden but there was more to it than met the eye, partly because it was arranged on several levels, with little terraces against the wall at the back. In the left hand corner there was a small cobbled area, and in the middle of this was a pond shaped like a star. If you turned a tap in the kitchen the fountain came on — tiny arcs of water shooting out of a little lead pipe at each corner and meeting in the middle. Behind the pond was a roofed-in area that had probably been built as a summerhouse, but which we used to store garden tools. All over the roof, and indeed all over the walls beside it, was growing the most wonderful rose. The name of it was Alberic Barbier, and in early summer it was completely covered in the most delicately scented cream-coloured flowers which my mother really loved. But apart from that the garden had been very neglected and she decided to fill it with flowers. She planted ferns and periwinkle in the shady part, near the house, and she grew several fruit trees by simply burying the stones of any fruit she happened to be eating. One of these, a white-skinned Italian peach, grew into a fine tree and produced huge amounts of fruit many years after she had died. But we needed more flowers, and shortly after we moved in we had an idea where we could get some. In Hammersmith, just up the road, a whole terrace of houses was being knocked down to make way for a new flyover. We had noticed, on our walks up to Hammersmith Broadway, that the houses had rather nice gardens. So when the people had moved out and the builders had moved in, we began a series of night-time raids. We would dress up in dark clothes, and we would take our buckets and garden tools and let ourselves into the gardens, now backed with rather sad, broken houses. In the half-light of the distant street lamps we would dig and scrabble and remove anything that looked faintly promising. She may have been green fingered, but my mother did not know a great deal about flowers so we usually had no idea what we were getting, and in any case we couldn't see. But they all got shoved into the garden at Lower Mall and soon it was full of glorious surprises, including many of Sophie's favourites, peonies and sweet williams.

9 Lower Mall would prove, in the event, to be an extremely unlucky house, and our lives certainly became more troubled after we moved there. But at first it all seemed idyllic. It was such a beautiful place to live. Because there was no road in front, just the towpath, it was very quiet, with only the hum of traffic going over the bridge and the river noises. It was the

river that made it so perfect. There it was, just on the other side of the wall opposite, where the great catalpa, or indian bean, tree grew. When the tide was up it slopped against the wall and if you looked at it from above there was always a most fascinating mixture of debris, mainly old bits of wood, which shifted around constantly like a kaleidoscope — a whole ribbon of it in a wide stripe alongside the wall. And when the tide went out there was the brown river mud in a huge bank, thick and shiny and bumpy, with a ribbon of water sliding down the middle under the bridge. Then there were the boats. Barges, motor boats, people practising rowing in ones or twos or eights, the river police — every one that went by left a wake and made the water at high tide splash and slop wildly against the wall. At night, the lights on the bridge were reflected in the water and they sparkled and twinkled and made changing wave patterns on the ceilings of the rooms at the front of the house.

We all loved the river. Percy, who for a short time had a flat on the second floor, bought a little boat with a petrol motor which she kept at the boatyard a little further along the Mall. The boatyard was great. It had a notice up at the entrance with a picture of a skull and crossbones and a sign saying 'Trespassers will be Drowned', and once you had clambered over the gate in the wall, there was a maze of rafts, with little boats of all kinds tied up to them, bobbing about. In truth I did not like Percy's boat much because the smell of the petrol engine made me sea-sick, but I did get onto the river even so, in my very own boat, which my father bought me for a birthday present. This was a little clinker-built rowing boat, solid and sturdy, and we were allowed to moor it to a raft outside the Blue Anchor pub nearby. So I took to the water, which was quite a scary experience, as I had not realised how strong the tide would be. The first time I took the boat out I went with the tide and ended up in Putney in a flash, then spent the whole of the rest of the day rowing back again, my arms almost out of their sockets from the effort. After that I was more careful, and the boat gave me many hours of pleasure until one boat-race day it was ripped off its mooring by the huge waves made by the river traffic, carried down the river and smashed into firewood.

This was not the end of my adventures on the river. I could also go out in a canoe, with my new friends who lived on Chiswick Mall, just a short walk away. They were the Lousadas, and we soon became really good friends with them. The mother and father were Anthony and Jocelyn, and my parents had known Jocelyn for a long time because, as Jocelyn Herbert, she had been a design student at the London Theatre Studio before the war. They lived in a big house, not an old one but one which seemed to suggest wealth without being at all ostentatious. There were books everywhere, huge sofas, old rugs on the floors, dressers of beautiful china in the kitchen. (I once managed to break a cup belonging to a priceless set that Antony had given Jocelyn for her birthday — she was very nice about it but I felt terrible). They had four children. Sandra, the eldest, a big, jolly, attractive teenager, was source of wonder to me as I would sometimes catch sight of her kissing her boyfriends in what seemed to me a frighteningly erotic way. Jenny, two years older then me, was the one I loved and admired the most. She was imaginative, original, artistic, and made me feel very pedestrian and dull by comparison. Then there were the twins, Julian and Olivia, a bit younger than I was and attractive little round things who were fun to play with.

Our social life really took off when we moved to into this circle. I played with the Lousada children frequently, though I was never sure whether in fact they really liked me all that much, and my parents joined in all the lunch parties and dinner parties — there always seemed to be something going on at the Lousadas. They had interesting friends, people like Arthur Koestler, and Laurie Lee with his beautiful big blonde wife Cathy. There was always plenty of good food, lots of wine, people sitting around talking and laughing. Further down Chiswick Mall, almost at the end, lived another family we saw sometimes, the Redgraves. Vanessa I was very much in awe of, as she seemed much older than I was and so very tall and beautiful. Corin was older too and for a brief period I thought him rather attractive in a blond and handsome sort of way, but I soon started to find him a bit cool and slightly dull. Lyn Redgrave was the same age as I was and she was quite good fun. Like me, she was a bit chubby, and her father never appeared to be very nice to her, apparently because of this, which seemed a bit unfair. I never got to know Michael at all well, but his wife Rachel Kempson appeared to me to be perfect. She smelled absolutely wonderful — my mother told me that this was because she had a special scent made for her at a place called Floris, and this wafted into the room before she did. When she hugged you she felt almost impossibly soft and sweet and her scent enveloped you like a fog. She was warm and beautiful and I always loved seeing her.

The high point of life on Chiswick Mall was the Christmas carol singing. This was no ordinary event. Everyone gathered at the Lousadas and practised a bit round the piano and then set off to entertain the neighbours. Michael Redgrave was always there: he had a terrific voice and was obviously glad of a chance to show it off. Accompanying the voices was an oboe, played by Julian Trevelyan, a painter who lived with his painter wife Mary a little further down the Mall. This all sounds impossibly Dickensian and altogether too good to be true, and in the end it turned out to be just that. But the dark underside did not appear straight away.

Soon after we moved to Lower Mall my parents got involved in a production of Ibsen's *Hedda Gabler*. Percy and my mother designed the sets and costumes, and George acted in it, and later took over the direction too. He played George Tesman, the husband of Hedda, who was played by my godmother Peggy. Rachel Kempson was also in it, and so was Michael Macliammoir, an actor from Ireland who we had never met before and who became a really good friend. Although it transferred later to the West End, *Hedda Gabler* started out on tour and then played at the Lyric Hammersmith,

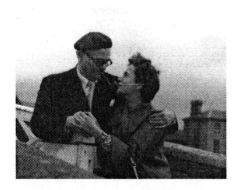

*George and Peggy on tour with* Hedda Gabler

which was less than ten minutes walk from our new house. It was one of those productions that seem just to go right, especially after George took over the direction from Peter Ashmore. The intention of the designers and the director was to set this powerful, brooding tragedy in light, Scandinavian decor, and to emphasise the comic aspects of the play. They rather overdid this attempt at first, and the audience at the first tryout, in Dublin, roared with laughter throughout. But after they had toned down the comic business the play was hugely successful. The company became like a family, and because we were so close by we saw a great deal of all the actors.

For me it was a time of great closeness to my father. My mother was out working a great deal, overseeing the costumes for *Hedda* as well as for an opera called *Nelson* which opened at Sadlers Wells a couple of weeks later, but George was at home a good deal. I helped him to learn his lines, something I loved to do, reading the other parts to give him the cues for his own lines: 'Think of that, Hedda dear!'. Once the play had opened he would always be at home for his tea before the show, and I used to cook it for him. Almost every evening he would have a boiled egg (with an Energen Roll), and we worked out a system of timing it by my heartbeats — a rather cumbersome process, as I had to stand by the cooker with my hand pressed against my heart, counting for three and a half minutes. I could have used the clock but it would not have been such fun.

Peggy Ashcroft was an excellent godmother to me, as she took her role very seriously. She always gave me birthday presents, often very good ones. I think it was for my twelfth birthday that she gave me a set of records of Mozart's *Eine Kleine Nacht Musik*, a piece of music that absolutely enchanted

68

me — I used to sit in my room playing it ceaselessly. This introduction to Mozart no doubt paved the way for my passion for *The Magic Flute* a year or so later. My father and Percy worked on a production of the opera at Sadlers Wells and I became obsessed with it, playing it on records over and over again while I read the libretto.

All my childhood we were on very good terms with Peggy and often used to visit her and her family in their lovely house in Hampstead. Her husband Jeremy Hutchinson, twinkly and funny, was a barrister, and her two children were close to my age, Eliza a little older and Nicky a little younger. They used to have the most wonderful parties, everything glittering and warm and beautiful and opulent. Peggy was really adorable, warm and pretty and charming, and she always made me feel welcome and loved whenever I visited her, right into my adulthood. When I was little I had no idea of the subtext of her marriage, but it was during the *Hedda* period, soon after we had moved to Lower Mall, that I found out.

I can still remember the day with absolute clarity. My mother and I had gone out for a walk along the river, and had ended up at the place known as the Green, an open area just before the pub called the Dove, which was next to William Morris's house. It was a fine day, with lots of people around. And it was on the Green, for some reason that I have completely forgotten, that she suddenly told me that Peggy and Tony Britton had been having an affair, which had by that time come to an end though Peggy was still 'very much in love with him'.

This information was a terrible shock to me. Not that it had escaped my notice that married people had affairs. In the theatre it was going on around us all the time, people getting married, getting divorced, living together, breaking up, with monotonous regularity, so that my parents' marriage often seemed the only stable one I could think of. But this news was like being hit on the head and in the heart, with two simultaneous blows. Peggy, who I had always seen as such a close unit with Jeremy, whose children I was friends with, who was almost family: this was bad enough. But

*Peggy and Tony Britton in* The Merchant of Venice *at Stratford, at the time of their love affair*

Peggy and Tony Britton — Tony Britton with whom I had been for more than a year desperately, powerfully, painfully in love! How could I deal with this information? However, when I had time to process it, it did explain a lot, especially my father's attitude to Tony Britton. But I would never be able to love Tony B quite so much again.

I suppose that one reason for my mother's sudden decision to confide in me was connected with the fact that I was being seen, and treated, rather more like a grown-up person when we moved to Lower Mall. Christina had left us and no-one came to replace her, so when my parents were working I was left pretty much to my own devices, which would prove to have rather devastating results not long afterwards.

And my parents were working, if anything, harder than ever. In addition to all the plays and films Sophie was doing, this was the time when she re-started the Motley couturier house that she had run so successfully in the late '30s. This time some financial assistance came from Monty Berman, of Berman's, the famous theatrical costumiers with whom my mother had had a long professional relationship. She managed to rent some premises over a restaurant in St Martin's Lane: ironically, these were directly opposite where the old Motley studio had been before it was bombed in the war. Because the Motley dress shop had gone bankrupt before the war, she could not use the

Motley name for the collections, and for some reason decided to use the name Elizabeth Curzon. Hilda Reader, the superb cutter who had been recruited by the Motleys from Hayes village in 1932, was employed full-time to oversee the making of the dresses, and for a limited period the venture seemed to be a great success.

My mother's designs were unlike anything that anyone else at the time was doing. One of her favourites, and mine too, was a dress made entirely from cotton curtain-lace, cream-coloured, thick and heavy, with beautiful coarse patterns all over it — a huge skirt and a tight little bodice. Another one, very striking and often photographed, was made of

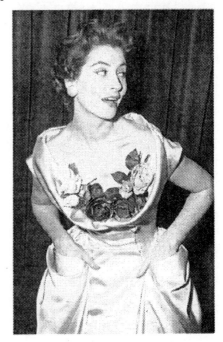

*Eliabeth Curzon couturier dress*

heavy satin, with a long full skirt. It had a sort of swag at the low neckline made from a drape of satin, and inside the swag was an arrangement of fake flowers, which somehow managed to lie elegantly around the model's lovely décolletage. I became fascinated by fashion at this time and used to spend hours cutting out pictures of beautifully dressed ladies from *Vogue* and *Harper's Bazaar*, which I was allowed to stick all over the walls of the downstairs lavatory at Lower Mall. Soon the whole room was completely papered with exquisite creatures like greyhounds, with tiny waists and little hats perched on top of smooth hairdos, and skirts swooping outwards over long legs and spindly high heels.

I also loved to go to the fittings at Elizabeth Curzon. I could sit for hours watching the ladies trying on their dresses. Sometimes they were people I knew, actresses like Rachel Kempson, but there were also very grand society ladies and even aristocrats. Probably the grandest customer of all was the Duchess of Argyll, who had several dresses made for her. Tall and elegant, not as young as she had been, she would swoop in for her fittings from time to time and for these I had to go and sit with the cutters and seamstresses. But my mother told me that, because the Duchess had been a famous beauty and was obsessed with keeping her looks, she never smiled or frowned, in order to keep her face from getting wrinkled. This always sounded very difficult to keep up — we tried to do it and succeeded for about three minutes at the most. Perhaps she did smile in the presence of her peers, but she certainly did not smile at her dressmaker.

The high point of the Elizabeth Curzon era was a wonderful dress-show, which took place in some large West-End restaurant. Little gilt chairs were laid out along a runway, and there were curtains at the end behind which the models could change. The most important and successful models of the day were hired for it, people like Barbara Goolen and Fiona Campbell-Walter. Some famous actor or other was the compere, and a cousin of my mother's played the piano. Her name was Anne Maurice, and she was French, or half-French. I remember being rather impressed as I had heard of her daughter, who was a newly successful actress, Virginia McKenna. I was hoping she would come to the show, but she did not, and to this day I have never met her, although I like to tell people when her films appear on television that she is my distant cousin. The show seemed to be a success, and Elizabeth Curzon always seemed busy, but for some reason it folded and Sophie went back to concentrating just on theatre, opera and films.

# 6

Although in retrospect I believe my father was getting a bit restless and unhappy by the time we moved out of Addison Road, I don't think I was aware of it at the time. We still seemed to be functioning as a family just as well as we ever did. As well as the holidays in France, we would go out together, often to see plays or dance performances or films, sometimes for meals at one of my father's favoured French restaurants in Soho. It was on one such outing that I met a cousin of my father's, who we encountered quite by chance in the West End. His name was Harry Carpos, and he was about my father's age, looking like a swarthier and more untrustworthy version of George. He wore an overcoat with an astrakhan collar – what Sophie called an actor-manager's coat. My father greeted him fairly coolly, and after a rather stilted conversation we parted. Then he told us the history of his prior knowledge of this rarely met first cousin.

George loved to tell stories about his rather curious forebears. So I knew a lot already about my great-grandfather Henry Devine, born in Dublin in 1839, who had moved to Manchester and married the daughter of his Greek employer. She was Cariclia Couvelas, born in Constantinople in 1841 to a family from the island of Khios, which lies just off the Turkish coast. How was her English? Not recorded. Did Henry learn some Greek? Quite probably, since he removed himself to Greece sometime in the last decades of the nineteenth century. With him went his wife, his elder daughter (another Cariclia, born in 1864) and his younger, Helena, and Pericles, the baby of the family, who grew up to be a sad and sickly youth with a drooping moustache. Four more sons, including my grandfather Georgios, stayed behind in England. The family settled in Athens, where Mrs Devine died, the girls married, and Pericles succumbed to tuberculosis. By this time old Irish Henry had taken to religion, though not the brand of high Anglicanism practised by his son Minos, who became a pillar of the church in London. Henry became a member of the Plymouth Brethren, an unrelenting sect of Evangelicals, and spent his final days as an itinerant preacher in the hill villages above Athens. The whole family seems to have become Plymouth Brethren, and Cariclia and Helena remained so after their marriages.

Now George filled in some of the gaps. Harry Carpos was the son of one or other of these two aunts: more likely perhaps Helena, since Cariclia would have been in her late forties at least by the presumed time of Harry's birth. My father had had little or no contact with him since their first meeting many years before, when sixteen-year-old Harry had been sent to England for a visit. George, meeting his cousin at the station, had been encouraged by the sight of a violin tucked under his arm.

*Oh, you play the violin! What do you play?*
*Hymns* (in a heavy Greek accent).

Predictably, Harry had rebelled violently against his repressive upbringing, and a few years later was reported to have fled the fold and to be living a life of extreme dissipation, indulging long-suppressed desires for wine, women and whatever else accompanied them. When we met him in London he looked seedy but prosperous, like a man whose money has been made in ways of which he is not altogether proud. But I never did find out exactly what those ways had been.

Although Lower Mall had not been terribly expensive to buy, my parents could not afford to live there without a lodger. In any case, there was already a self-contained flat on the top floor, which had been added to the house at some time in the 1930s and which had been designed by a famous architect called Maxwell Frye. The flat was indeed very 1930s, with big sliding windows going the whole width of the house and looking out over the river. It had a huge L-shaped studio room, a tiny galley kitchen and bathroom and a sort of non-area of a lower roof where steps led up to the roof proper, a flat affair with railings where we used to stand to watch the Boat Race every year, cheering on Oxford since my father had been there. In fact everyone we knew seemed to have been there including the lodger who moved into the flat. He was Tony Richardson, who we had met when he had directed George in the Chekov television play and who was now fully engaged in working with him on the renewed Royal Court scheme.

Tony seemed to me to be the tallest person I had ever met, skinny and slightly stooping, and ridiculously extravagant in voice, gesture, and attitude. He moved in with a flatmate, a satanically handsome American sociologist called George Goetschius. My father had a rather nervous and mistrustful attitude to homosexuality, which was ironic since almost everyone who worked for him at the Royal Court was engaged in it to a greater or lesser degree, and possibly he did not realise, at least at first, that George and Tony were anything other than friends. I'm sure Sophie knew they were lovers, and Cathy and I, by now very sophisticated, strongly suspected it. But Tony, in any case, liked women as well as men. For a time, soon after he moved in, he was desperately in love with an Australian actress called Diane Cilento, a beautiful blonde with a wonderful husky voice. She tormented him endlessly.

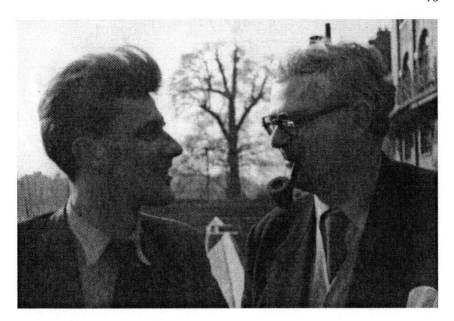

*Tony and George on Lower Mall*

One day she turned up in a huge fur coat, and revealed soon afterwards that she was completely naked beneath it. However her nakedness was not for Tony, but apparently just intended to increase his desperation, which it did. 'I must have her', he would howl to my mother, but all to no avail.

Apart from Diane and the theatre, what Tony really loved was birds and reptiles. He bought strange silver grass snakes, which he released onto the lawn in the back garden, where they used to lurk about and suddenly slither out. We hated and feared them but Tony loved them and used to pick them up and watch them for hours as they twisted about his hands. He also liked to pick up and caress the toads with which he had peopled the pond. Sophie used to say he was a cold-blooded creature himself and that was why he loved them all so much. More than anything else, though, he had a passion for birds. Almost every Saturday morning he would persuade Sophie to take him down to Shepherd's Bush market, where there were numerous shops full of little caged birds for sale. They would walk down the market arm in arm (a strange sight as he was about a foot taller than she was) and each time they came near to one of the bird shops she would feel him start to tremble violently from the excitement of it all. Sometimes he would buy a couple of birds, which at first he kept in cages in the studio. Soon however he decided to build them an aviary, and glassed over the lower roof area where he then could set them free to fly and perch and twitter to their hearts' content.

I don't think either my mother or I ever felt quite comfortable with Tony, but he could be incredibly kind when he was in the mood. A year or so after we had moved to Lower Mall, when I had been sent to boarding school, he did two things which were large, unforgettable and rather wonderful gestures. First of all, not long after I had arrived at the school, I was lonely, unhappy and above all hungry. I hated the food, and craved for chocolate. One day I had the idea of writing to Tony to see if he would send me a bar or two. But a bar or two would have been a little tame for Tony, so he got hold of a huge cardboard box, took it to the sweet shop on the corner, and had it filled completely to the brim with every kind of chocolate there was in the shop. When it arrived at school it made everyone very astonished, and very friendly, and made me a good deal fatter than I already was.

The other thing he did was also very amazing. I had been lamenting the fact that Valentine's day was coming and I was sure that I would be the only person in my class without a card. But when the day arrived, instead of one card, there were three for me. All were quite different, all were signed with cryptic messages, and one had a black thumbprint on it as it was, supposedly, from the coal-man. My credit went up hugely as a result, but I was not fooled for long, and realised that Tony must have sent them. It was, though, a kind gesture and I was grateful to him for it.

I was never quite sure how Tony felt about my mother, trips to the bird-shops notwithstanding. I always believed he had encouraged my father to leave her, and I was quite surprised to find, when his autobiography appeared, that he had nothing at all negative to say about her. But I think they had quite a good relationship in the very early days, and it must have been then that occurred the memorable and funny episode of the dog impersonation. What happened was this. My mother was exhausted after a long week of work, but she wanted to go upstairs and see Tony and George. As she reached the third flight of stairs, the steep ones that led up to the flat, fatigue got the better of her and she started to go up on her hands and knees. At the moment when she got to the top, the studio door opened and an ankle emerged. Naturally enough, she started growling loudly and took a snapping bark at it. Unfortunately Tony and George were not alone: they had some rather grand visitors, middle-class American relatives of George, who stood there in astonishment looking down at this little woman in a striped sailor's top pretending to be a small terrier. There was a long pause and then Tony said, 'This is my landlady'.

Within quite a short time of moving to Lower Mall the pattern of my life would change dramatically, and my world would be shattered by a large internal explosion. But this did not happen at once. Initially things went on much as they always had. I was still going to Miss Ironsides', taking the bus every day along from Hammersmith to Kensington, walking down the Gloucester Road. The Turners had moved, too, right over to the other side of London where they had bought a wonderful, huge, house in Highgate where Coleridge had once lived. But Cathy and I were still best friends — perhaps even closer than ever. Not terribly happy at home, rather disharmonious with both her mother and her eldest brother, she would spend many of her free days with us at Lower Mall. One day she and I devised a game that proved to be surprisingly successful. We got some empty bottles with good corks, and we painstakingly wrote out messages, which we put inside, sealed up, and cast into the river. The messages began like this:

*We are two ladies in distress*
*9 Lower Mall (Hammersmith, London, W6) is our address.*
*With our tutor harsh and cruel*
*Our lovers dear did fight a duel...*

The gist of the whole thing was that we were waiting to be rescued, but I'm not sure how seriously we believed that anything would ever come of it. Imagine our surprise when one day, well over a year later, a letter came from Belgium with a finely poetic reply. A covering letter explained that our bottle had been found by an old fisherman who had taken it to his local village schoolmaster for a translation. Intrigued, the schoolmaster had sent the response. Even better, some months later I was as usual hanging over the balcony watching the passers-by when a dapper, foreign-looking young man came by and accosted me: on investigation he proved to be the very schoolmaster who had written the letter, on holiday in London and curious to see the writers of the appealing poem. He came in for a cup of tea, but whether he had been expecting a real damsel in distress or not we never found out.

We also continued to spend summer holidays at Stratford, sometimes accompanied by Cathy. Life there was very sweet, and there seemed to be so many things to enjoy. Sometimes there would be cricket matches between teams composed of the actors and other staff. Percy was a tremendous wicket keeper and spent a lot of the game crouched behind the wickets, looking very fine in her white clothes. Peggy Ashcroft, rather surprisingly, used to bowl quite well, and one day in a practice session before the game she narrowly avoided killing me by sending a very fast and injudicious ball whizzing in my direction.

Some of the best times were those I spent with Peggy's family at their rented home in Alveston, a huge white house with enormous lawns stretching down to the river, large airy rooms, and a feeling of peace and opulence. I

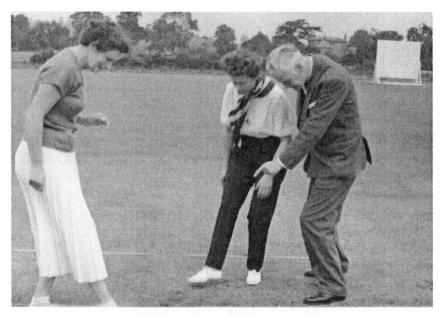

*Cricket at Stratford. Peggy, Glen and Barbara Jefford inspect the pitch.*

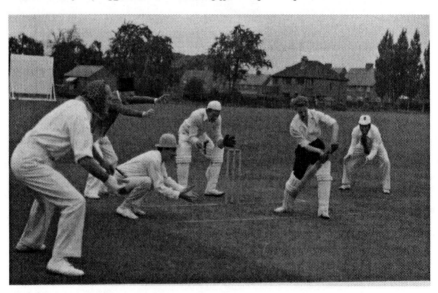

*Cricket at Sratford: from left, Harry Andrews, Glen, unidentified, Tony Britton, Rachel Kempson, unidentified*

got on well with Eliza and Nicky, though often I seemed to set them off into uncontrollable giggles. I remember one day in particular when their tiny Scottish nanny took us into Stratford to do some shopping. Somehow or other, in one shop, I managed to say something which started us all laughing so much we were nearly sick with it, and were thrown out of the shop onto the pavement where we continued to wheeze and shriek, in spite of the staring passers-by. Nanny, meanwhile, was trying to be cross but seemed in danger of joining in.

Alveston, where Peggy lived, was also the place where you could go punting. That was something Sophie and I really enjoyed doing. We would go and hire a boat for the afternoon and set off in the opposite direction to the town. The river was really quiet down here, just smooth slippery black water and willow trees. You could go for miles without meeting anyone, and it was a good place to practice. I got rather good at it, dipping and swinging the pole, the water running down my arm. All the actors enjoyed punting when they had breaks from rehearsals, so you could and sometimes did meet people you knew — with luck, someone you were in love with. I had stopped loving Tony Britton after my mother's terrible revelation, but I soon found others to replace him, even if not quite so intensely. Laurence Harvey was one: I was struck by his elegance and beauty, and loved his curious voice with its combination of Lithuanian and South African accents. I do not think he ever knew I existed, but I admired him for months and even experienced a brief revival of the same feeling three years later when he played Horner in *The Country Wife* at the Royal Court. I never saw him punting, but I did see Keith Michell, another rather brief passion of mine. Occasionally there would be an after-theatre punting party. Angela Baddeley, Glen's wife, liked to arrange these. People would set off after the show, taking the punts from the landing stages near the theatre, and drift down with candles in jars, champagne, various kinds of food, and moor somewhere outside the town to eat and drink and sing late into the night.

I was allowed to come to these parties. In fact in theory I was allowed to come to all the parties, including the ones which were invariably held after the first nights. I enjoyed them, though no one much ever talked to me. I just used to dart about, picking at the food, watching people, listening in to conversations. I say in theory because on one memorable occasion I almost didn't get to go. I can't remember which play had just opened, but I know Cathy had been staying with us and both of us had been taken by my mother to see the first night. Afterwards there was to be a party at Glen and Angela's pretty house. Sophie and I and Cathy drove there in our terrible old Austin, parked, and went up to the front door. Sophie rang the bell. When the door opened, Angela was there in her best party dress, a welcoming smile on her face, which disappeared as she caught sight of us. 'Oh my God, you haven't brought those two ghastly girls!', she said. But there we were. I rarely saw my mother angry, but this was one occasion when I did. She didn't say much but she was really furious and Angela could see that she was. So she let us in, rather grudgingly, and the two of us sat on the sofa feeling unbelievably uncomfortable and out of place as Sophie socialised and chatted for enough time to make whatever point she felt it necessary to make.

I suppose I must have been bored sometimes at Stratford but I don't have any memory of this. The year I was thirteen I was actually given a job to do — a paid one, too — helping to sell souvenir programmes in the foyer during the matinees. I enjoyed doing it but most of all I enjoyed the sense that I was doing something that a grown-up person would normally do, and I felt intensely proud.

It was at Stratford, when I was twelve, that I ended up in hospital having my appendix out. I had been complaining of intermittent stomach aches, not particularly bad ones, but annoyingly recurrent. Eventually the doctor said it would do no harm to take my appendix out. The hospital was rather sweet and old-fashioned — what they call a cottage hospital, with long wooden huts surrounded by neat little gardens. An appendix operation was far from serious, I was told, and I was led to expect a tiny little scar. But when I came round from the anaesthetic, I found I had a huge long stripe all down the side of my stomach. The doctors said it was just as well they had operated when they did as my appendix was in a really bad state and had been about to burst: the long opening was so that they could get it out more easily in its swollen and infected state. Instead of stitches I had metal clips holding it together and it hurt quite a lot when, ten days later, they took them out and clinked them one at a time into a metal bowl. Then I was allowed to go home which made me happy, as I had felt very bored and trapped in the hospital, even though I had had a stream of visitors and had been allowed to totter into the garden in my dressing gown. Because I had been so bored, my mother decided to take me out on the river next day, and we hired a rowing boat. I loved rowing and persuaded her to let me have a go, but the physical effort proved to be too much for my scar which started to pop open a bit. We both panicked, having visions of the whole thing opening right up like a faulty zip and letting my entire inside fall out into the bottom of the boat. But when we raced back to the hospital they assured us this couldn't happen, and told us off for over-exertion. It would be fine, they said, and so it was, except that at the base of my long scar I have a little circular extension, a token of the day we rowed on the Avon in the sunshine.

How we used to laugh sometimes, my mother and I. Not at anything in particular, or at least not at anything which seems remotely funny in retrospect. But sometimes one of us would set the other off and we would be weak with giggles in no time at all. One day I remember clearly going for a stroll in the field on the opposite side of the river from the theatre. It was rather a boring field, full of dogs going to the lavatory and people wandering about in a rather desultory way. You could get across there on a little ferry, which was really the whole point of the expedition. Right in the middle of the field was a little dilapidated wooden hut, a disused snack stall. Over the boarded up window, it had a sign, and the sign said: 'Tea, Ices and'. For some reason this started us off, and quite soon we were unable to continue to walk. We had to lie down on the grubby grass nearby, crying with desperate laughter.

Meanwhile, back in London, my father and Tony had finally managed to get the English Stage Company at the Royal Court off the ground. This was a tremendously exciting time for all of us. Above all, because my whole family and everyone else we knew seemed to be involved, there was a great sense of communal endeavour, in the very early days at least. Sophie and Percy designed all the early productions and I was allowed to come to all

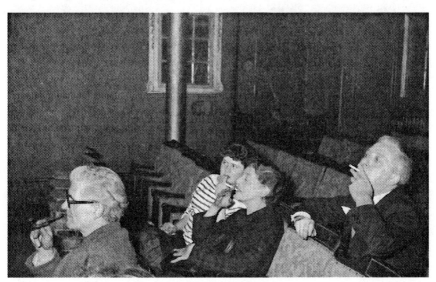

*In the stalls at a run-though of* The Mulberry Bush, *George, me, Sophie and Angus Wilson*

the rehearsals. I was even roped in, being asked by George to make some EXIT signs to hang over the doors in the auditorium, which I tried to do with bits of cardboard and poster paints. They were not up to scratch, not surprisingly since I was only thirteen and not a graphic artist. But it was kind of him to ask.

The most exciting bit was looking for the new plays. Finding new writers was the whole point of the English Stage Company: it was a Writers' Theatre.

This was in fact my father's great departure from the footsteps of Michel Saint Denis. In other ways his ideas still were rooted in Michel's pre- and post-war teaching: the simplicity, the lack of illusion, everything honest and stripped down to basics. But finding new writers was a new departure, and a challenge. Advertisements were put in *The Stage*, novelists were approached to see if they would like a change of direction. Angus Wilson responded to that appeal and in the event his play, *The Mulberry Bush*, became the first production at the Court. But for a really unknown name the public had to wait for the fourth production, the one that really shot the Court into notoriety: *Look Back in Anger.*

The whole story of the finding of *Look Back* has been mythologised, and I can't add much to what has already been said. But I do remember that my father and Tony were really excited. The advertisements seem to have produced nothing much that was worth having — I know myself from a year as Literary Manager at the Court after my father died that there is a lot of dross out there — a lot of people who think they can write and whose depressing proofs to the contrary seem to land monotonously often on one's desk. So when *Look Back* plopped through the letter-box it was greeted with intense delight. The first thing that happened was that we had to meet the writer. Oddly enough, John Osborne turned out to be living just down the road, on a barge which was moored on Chiswick Mall, within sight almost of the Lousadas' house. The boat was not his — it belonged to his friend Anthony Creighton, and he was living there because he was completely broke. They were an unprepossessing couple, both in rather shabby blue blazers with tarnished gilt buttons, but they quickly came to be regular visitors at Lower Mall. Although John was supposedly heterosexual, and indeed went through strings of wives, I had the strongest of impressions that he and Anthony were lovers. I have to say that I never really grew to like John, but he did have an enormous amount of some kind of charisma. In those early days, before he got sleek and successful, he seemed to sparkle despite the shabby clothes and the rather pugnacious attitude.

*Look Back* was to be Tony's production, but although John and Tony continued to have a working partnership John developed the greatest and most sincere of loves for George, who was possibly the only person he managed to care for genuinely. My father, meanwhile, was involved in productions of varying degrees of success. Acting as well as directing, he gave a marvellous performance as Judge Danforth in Arthur Miller's *The Crucible*, and later in the first season a grotesquely satirical depiction of a priest, Father Golden Orfe, in Nigel Dennis's *Cards of Identity*. But it was directing and running the theatre that took up most of his time. Early in the season he did a production of two verse plays by Ronald Duncan, mainly because Duncan was involved with the Board of the English Stage Company. So George was doing the plays out of a sense of duty, and his lack of enthusiasm really showed in the final result, which was so resoundingly unsuccessful that they plays came off after only eight performances.

The good thing that came out of the Duncan plays was a friendship between my parents and the talented painter who had been employed to design them. His name was John Minton, and we all came to love him very much. Homosexual, alcoholic, neurotic in the extreme, he was one of the most charming, funny and sweet-natured people I have ever met. He absolutely adored my mother, and confided all his troubles to her endlessly. He not only presented my father with large and rather valuable canvasses, but he also took a liking to me and Catherine and gave us both framed water-colours to hang on our walls. Later that year, when I was away at boarding-school, he wrote me a letter that was absolutely enchanting — all written in green and purple ink, decorated in the margins with the most delightfully intricate pictures. I kept the letter for a long time, but somehow in the course of many moves it has been lost, something I shall never cease to regret.

It is sad to have to write that Johnny Minton's final tragedy was associated with the Court, and with my mother. At the Court there was a Master Carpenter whose name was Kevin Maybury. He was Australian, and was amazingly beautiful, tall, strong and blond.

I was much in love with him, and Cathy and I composed a song about him, which we sang to the tune of Nuts-in-May:

*All in the month of May-bury*
*When green buds are a-sway-bury*
*I mean to marry Maybury*
*I pray that he will stay by me.*
*I'll wash and bake and scrub and clean*
*Till nothing neater has been seen*
*Our house will be fit for a QUEEN*
*Or doctor, lawyer, judge or dean.*

A lot of emphasis was given to the 'Queen' in the penultimate line because, judging not only from his total lack of interest in us but also from other things we heard and saw, we began to wonder whether Kevin really liked women at all. Johnny Minton wondered this too, and he was, in fact, very soon dreadfully in love with him. He painted a portrait of him, which is now in the National Gallery, and he pined and pined because nothing seemed to be coming of it all. And then one evening, when I was away at school, my mother had a telephone call from Johnny, sounding very sad and desperate — could he come round and talk to her? But this was one of so many of such calls she had had from him, and she was deeply tired after a long week's work. 'I'll meet you tomorrow, darling', she said, as kindly as she could. Imagine how she must have felt when the news came next day that Johnny had committed suicide in his studio, seemingly only shortly after he had called on her for the help she didn't feel able to give. As everyone pointed out he probably would have done it anyway, sooner or later, but her shock and her self-blame were very great.

During that first season at the Court, Cathy and I were constantly hanging around the theatre — it was the following autumn that both of us finally disappeared to boarding-school. There was a great community feel to those early days — everyone gathering for meals in the London Transport café at the back of the theatre, where you could get a huge mug of blisteringly strong sweet tea and a plate of egg and chips for — well, whatever ludicrous- sounding sum things cost in those far-off days. Right behind the theatre was a row of tiny cottages which, when they were first acquired, became the wardrobe and scenery and property workshops. Always quite handy at making things, I was allowed to come in and help with the scene-painting, which was supervised by our friend and neighbour Jocelyn Lousada, and the prop-making. As usual Cathy and I spent a lot of time watching rehearsals and had a lot of fun making up poems about the actors, writers and designers. They were a new verse form which we had invented ourselves. Here are some examples:

*John*
*With nothing on*
*Osborne*
*Just like the day he was born.*

*Mary*
*Had a dairy*
*Ure*
*From which the milk was pure.*

*Kenneth*
*At his zenith*
*Haigh*
*Is awfully vague.*

The best ones, obviously, were the ones that seemed to have some relevance to the reality of the person concerned, but it did not really matter to us whether they did or not. They made us scream with laughter in any case.

So life in these early days of the Court seemed to be a great deal of fun. But it was at around this time that something happened which was to change everything I thought and felt about my life, and afterwards nothing would ever be the same. What happened was this. My father and Tony were mostly at the Court and my mother was working too, both there and elsewhere, so she was not at home much either, and I no longer had an au-pair. So when I was not hanging around the theatre I spent a good deal of time at home alone. I didn't mind this. I used to read a lot, and listen to music, and practise cooking. One place I enjoyed being very much was my father's study. It was on the second floor, right next to my room but at the back of the house — quite a small room, with a big alcove attached which he used as a library. On one side was the meccano theatre, still in use, and a huge radio which you could listen to French stations on. On top of the radio was the big white pottery bowl with all George's pipes in it, arranged neatly with their bowls hooked over the edge. But the main thing in the room was his desk, a large and rather fine mahogany affair with a morocco leather top. On top of the desk were papers, held down by his special paper weight, which was a wonderful crystal thing called a prism, which made the light shine through in rainbow colours. Usually there would be a book he was reading, too — one I remember clearly was called *Le Grand Meaulnes*. I didn't know what Meaulnes meant, and for some reason associated it with sand-dunes — it was years before I discovered that it was someone's name.

I would sit at the desk for hours, staring out of the window, listening to the radio, looking at the books. Then one day I decided to try opening the drawers. The top ones had all the usual things in them that you would expect to find in a desk: paper, pens and pencils, rubbers, paper-clips. Further down there was blank paper for writing on, various boring looking office-type things, accounts. But down at the bottom was a drawer that was always locked, and in one of the top drawers there was a key that looked as if it would fit.

Did I hesitate before unlocking that drawer? Did I feel guilty, daring, ashamed? I think more than anything I felt nervous and curious – thinking about it now I can recall my heart beating very fast. And I was right to feel all this because what was in the drawer turned out to be something very momentous: it is not too much to say that it turned my whole world upside down. What was in the drawer were letters. They were all written to my father, and all written by one person. That person was Jocelyn Lousada. I read them all. By now my heart was thumping and my head was whirling

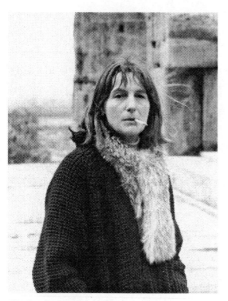

*Jocelyn in the early 1960s*

and I had no idea whether I was doing the wrong thing or not. In any case it was now far too late to turn back. Needless to say, they were love letters. Love letters of a very intense kind. Love letters from a person who is longing, craving to be with the person they were addressed to. And that person was my father, George Devine. One phrase in one letter got lodged in my mind and I wondered about it endlessly: 'Maybe someday our miracle will happen'.

By now I was so confused I didn't at all know what to do. I felt I could not talk to my mother about this as she might very well know nothing about it. But I did have one person I could tell — my dear friend Catherine. She was away at school by now, but we kept up an intense and frequent correspondence. So in the evening I sat in the sitting room with my writing pad and my pen and I started writing. The letter went on and on — there was so much to say. My mother was also in the room but I hardly noticed her, as I was so absorbed in writing the letter.

Then I had to go out of the room for some reason. I left the letter lying on the little coffee table. When I came back the first thing I saw was my mother's face, looking like I had never seen it look before. She had read the letter. The worst thing about this was the way I had told Catherine what had happened. I had written the whole thing in a sort of jocular tone, trying to show some sophistication about it all, to pretend that it was all OK and I could handle it, trying to be adult about it, trying to cover up my pain and shock. But my mother found this tone the most upsetting thing of all: she thought I had turned into a wicked, amoral sort of person who did not care about her or about what was happening in my father's life. What she did not tell me is whether she knew anything about it all before she read the letter and I feared deeply that she did not.

So secrets came out of the desk . I found out his and she found out mine. I was glad she had found out in one way because it was too big a burden for me to carry alone. But this created another burden for me. Now her unhappiness appeared to be my fault. When she became ill from cancer, which she did before too long, that was also my fault. I had opened the box and the bad things had flown out and messed up all our lives. Many people have assured me since that I was wrong, that she knew already and that the pain and shock she felt that day were a result of her feelings about me rather than of the discovery of the facts. But it is very difficult for children, and even for adults, not to take the blame, and it was a very long time before I was able to accept that I was not responsible for killing my mother.

# 7

Naturally enough, all my feelings about my life were radically altered by my discovery of Jocelyn's letters. After the first shock of reading my own letter to Cathy had died down, my mother tried to talk to me about it all, but really that did not help much. She was in so much pain herself that she couldn't find any way of easing mine. George never said a word. And I just felt as if I had grown up very quickly into a hard world where nothing was what it seemed and no one could be happy any more. Or at least that was what I felt at first. As time went on, I just accepted the situation and tried to get on with my life. I had to watch my mother getting thinner and sadder, but with an adolescent's selfishness I tried to distance myself as much as possible. I didn't want to be swamped by her grief.

These were internal changes. But externally my life changed too. Now this was all out in the open, my father started, very very slowly, to change the pattern of his life with us. The first thing he did was to move out of my mother's bedroom and into the rather cold extension which was at the back of the house: Sean Kenny, a designer friend of theirs, did the alterations to make it habitable. And while they were about it, the second floor was converted into a separate flat: I think at the back of George's mind was the need to bring in extra income for my mother when or if he actually moved out. This meant that my bedroom had to move downstairs into the front room, which had previously been inhabited by Angela Baddeley's sister Siggy, an antique dealer. Luckily I really liked the room, which had a little Cosi-stove where you could burn wood in the winter. There was a venetian blind on the window which didn't quite reach to the bottom and one morning as I was dressing I saw a man bent double outside the window watching me through the gap.

So began the long slow process of my father's going. It would be years before he finally left – first the move to a new room, then the curious arrangement of spending his weeks with Jocelyn and his weekends with us and finally, some three or four years later, the last move to Rossetti Studios for a new life with Jocelyn. But this was far in the future at this time.

If moving around the house was not enough, even more sweeping external changes awaited me. Now I was going to be sent to boarding school. This announcement followed quite quickly in the wake of the discovery of the letters, and was, I imagine, a direct result although it was not presented to me in that way. It was not meant to be a punishment, but it certainly felt like one. I think my parents must have felt that it was not good for me to be spending so much time alone, and I was too old for au pairs and nannies by then. Also, on another level, they were going through a gruelling emotional time and probably thought the atmosphere in the house would be hard for me to take. Not that they quarrelled — they never did, at least when I was around. I never heard them so much as raise their voices to each other in all my whole life with them. But my mother's pain was a reproach worse than any she could have screamed aloud, and my father's guilt made him react with impatience and irritation. He acted dismissively now, as if she was stupid, and when someone does that to you you instantly become stupid.

So, looked at like that, getting away probably wasn't such a bad thing. But I felt as if I was being expelled from my home and my family. And I hated being at boarding school, even though the place where I ended up certainly had its interesting and amusing side. The name of the school was Langford Grove. Essentially just a big Victorian house in lovely grounds, with a river, surrounded by fields, it was on the edge of a tiny village called Barcombe Mills, near Lewes in Sussex. The school had been running since the 1930s — I discovered many years later that Jocelyn had once been a pupil there, which I'm sure my mother did not know. In the thirties when the school had begun it had been big and successful, full of the children of famous artists and writers, but by the time I got there it had become a shadow of its former self. The classes were tiny, only about nine or ten girls in each, and the teaching was patchy, to say the least.

The school revolved entirely around its founder and headmistress, whose name was Elizabeth Curtis. We were to call her Mrs Curtis, but we called her Curty behind her back. She was ancient, or seemed so to us, though perhaps she was only in her sixties, and she was without doubt a true eccentric. Tall, with long grey hair that showed signs of having been red and which was caught together in a very untidy bun at the back, she wore floaty and trailing clothes and invariably a long string of beads around her neck. These she would twist around her fingers as she stood and talked to you, swaying gently from foot to foot as she did so, croaking at you in her curious parrot-like voice. She had strange eyes, which looked as if they were popping out of her head, and which Sophie told me were caused by something called a thyroid condition. She had been a sort of fringe member of the Bloomsbury group in the 1930s, when Vanessa Bell and Duncan Grant's daughter Angelica Bell had been a pupil at the school. Her granddaughter Lucinda, who became a good friend of mine, told me that when young she was noted for her flaming red hair, which used to stream behind her as she galloped over the Sussex Downs on a black stallion.

I said the teaching was patchy, but some of it was completely non-existent. We did not do any science at all, not even geography. In fact the only subjects we did, apart from art and drama which were hugely emphasised, were English, French, history and maths. Latin figured for a while, and I really loved it, but the Latin teacher got pregnant and left and no-one came to replace her. This was a pity as we had just got past something called the *Pons Asinorum* — the Bridge of Asses — so called because if you were an ass you could not get past it. I got past it alright because I was far from an ass. In fact I was quite clever and was put in a class with people a year older than I was, where I managed to get very good marks in most subjects without ever doing a stroke of work.

The work may have gone well, but my social life did not, at least at first. I was said to have what was called a strong character, which meant people either loved me or hated me, and some people definitely did hate me. The person who hated me the most, for reasons I never did discover, was called Harriet Llewellyn Jones. Perhaps it was something to do with our having the same name. One day she threw her hairbrush across the room and it hit me on the knee so hard that it got all puffy and swollen, a condition which was rather shamefully known as housemaid's knee. Another day she challenged me to a fight. This was a barbaric custom of long standing: two girls would have an arranged fight in front of the entire school, who never intervened but just allowed it to go on almost to the death. I thought the whole idea was extremely stupid, and when I was challenged I simply said no, I don't feel like it. This caused the most amazing shock waves as no one had ever refused to fight before. But interestingly enough my refusal broke the tradition entirely, and no one ever fought again.

There seemed to be, for some reason, a large number of aristocrats at the school. One was Elizabeth Keppel, who was the sister of the Marquis of Londonderry. Another, who became a good friend, had the wonderful name Everilda Dorothea Fleetwood Hesketh. Her family inhabited a manor house in the village of Hale, near Liverpool, and I was asked to stay there one holiday. My father was hugely amused by the double-barrelled name, by the whole upper-class thing. He laughed himself silly when I came home and revealed that I had been given ten shillings by Mrs Fleetwood Hesketh at the end of my stay — the joke was that usually it was the visitor who tipped the servants. When he eventually saw her which he did one day when we met the family somewhere unexpectedly, he was deeply disappointed: 'I thought she would look like a duchess but she looks like a charwoman'. She didn't, but I think he had imagined her dripping with diamonds. He always was rather an inverted snob.

I felt like a real misfit among all these upper-class girls. I felt very un-upper-class. I took refuge from it all in a very bad temper: something that had always been lurking but which had not until then had any real chance to express itself. I would give way to sudden rages at Langford, and scream and shout, sometimes rushing out of the classroom and hiding in the shrubbery until it passed. It actually frightened people sometimes and it certainly frightened me as it was a side of myself I didn't like to see at all. I was deep in adolescence, but the real trouble was that I was extremely unhappy and wanted to be at home. I missed my mother terribly and prayed every day that there would be a letter from her on the hall table after breakfast. There were often letters for me but not always from my mother although she was a good writer. Most of them, however, were from Cathy, who was away at boarding school too. We developed a system of writing to each other by return of post — not just a scribble, either, but long and closely written letters pouring out our hearts and minds. We stored them in the serving-hatch in the upstairs bathroom at Lower Mall in the holidays and they stayed there presumably for over twenty years until the flat was redecorated, and the letters vanished.

Because we had so few subjects to learn at Langford, we did manage to learn most of them very thoroughly. Not maths, though, or at least not as far as I was concerned. I was revolted by the maths teacher, an old man called Mr Haggart who was completely bald but had a long strip of greasy hair which he used to brush over the top of his head and which would slowly fall off during the lessons until it hung wispily over one shoulder. Everything about maths was dark to me, so much so that my parents were advised I would never get through O-level without private tuition. So off I went every week to Brighton, where I sat for an hour in a grubby bed-sit with a retired army major in a shabby blazer who chain-smoked and tried to explain to me the mysteries of geometry and algebra. His success can be measured by the fact that at the end of a year I sat the exam and got twenty per cent for it.

What we did do was plenty of art. In fact we spent one whole day a week doing that and nothing else. The art studio was a ramshackle black wooden building, more of a hut really, which sat in a wood down the garden. It was rather dark inside and so in fact not really ideal as a studio. But to compensate for the conditions, Curty did manage to get some very good teachers for us. She was a great patron of the arts and used to get real artists down from London to teach us. One was a painter called Edward Middleditch, who was very quiet and shy, and another was Frank Auerbach, young and foreign and dark, who was constantly exhorting us to 'put more paint on'. One day I went to an exhibition of his painting in London and saw how thick with paint his own canvasses were, and finally understood that he had wanted us to paint like he did. Then there was David Wynne, a sculptor, who was extremely suave and handsome. Many of the girls were in love with him but I was not, as I preferred actors.

Another subject that took up a lot of our time was drama. We had a teacher, Bertha Myers, who used to come down from London one day a week and who had been a student of my father's at the Old Vic School. I seemed to have some skill in acting and to get to play quite good parts. The most important was Falstaff in the *Merry Wives of Windsor*, in which my friend Lucinda Curtis played one of the wives. I had to have a padding for Falstaff, but I was rather well suited to the part as by this time I was really rather fat. The diet at the school did not help this at all. The food was vile but that simply meant you had to fill up on enormous slices of white bread and margarine with thin and tasteless mixed fruit jam spread on top. And sweets, hence my delight when Tony sent me the large quantities of chocolate. I was appalled one day to get on the scales in the matron's room and find I weighed ten and a half stone. For someone of five foot two-ish that was a lot, and I got teased for it, too. One day on the beach at Seaford I was struggling to change under an inadequate towel when two girls sitting near by said, very loudly, 'Look at her stomach — she's got great rolls of fat'. Unhappy though this made me, though, I simply ate more to cheer myself up.

One thing that did become clear when I was at Langford was how much of a non-conformist I was, and how little respect I had for rules and regulations. Refusing the fight was one example of this. Another time I shocked my class by pointing out to them that the teachers were, after all, simply human beings of a quite fallible kind, and that if they told us to do something and we did not want to do it, there was no way they could make us. This sounds pretty tame when you write it, but in fact it caused everyone to gaze at me in a sort of admiring horror. I was far from a rebel most of the time, as I didn't see the point of not doing what was prescribed. But I did put my ideas into practice a few times. One term, because I hated netball so much, I simply never went, and as we had a very high turnover in games mistresses the current one never even knew that I existed. On another occasion I was banished from an English lesson for talking in class. Everyone was reading *Paradise Lost*, and I didn't want to miss out on it because I really liked it. So after a minute or so I simply walked in and sat down again, and told the teacher I had decided to come back and hear what she had to say. I could tell that she was trying to look stern, but in fact she seemed to be trying not to laugh and she did let me stay.

Life at Langford was never exactly uneventful. One thing the school entirely lacked was any sense of justice. If Curty favoured you, all kinds of good things could and would happen, and if she did not you had a pretty miserable time. Part of the key to being liked was to be in favour with her beloved granddaughter Lucinda. During my eighteen months at the school, I was fortunately in Curty's favour, more or less, for a good deal of the time, but I did have a term when I was right out of it. You found out where you stood as soon as each new term started, as the place you had been put to sleep at night was the first and best indicator. There were two dormitories right next to Curty's drawing room, warm and cosy rooms where the elite slept. Then there were some in the middle which were fairly nondescript, and then there were a couple over the kitchen which were grim — cold and smelly — and in which I was unlucky enough to spend one term for reasons I have quite forgotten. The worst thing that happened that winter was that the pipes froze in the girls' bathrooms. For some reason they did not freeze in either Curty's rather grand bathroom or in the kitchen-man's appalling one. So we were divided sharply down the middle: those in favour bathed in Curty's bathroom, those out (including me) in the kitchen-man's black and greasy bath, looking over the yard where rats disported themselves among the dustbins. Having a bath in there probably made you dirtier than you were before you started but there was no arguing with Curty, who did not listen to complaints. In fact complaining would only make things worse.

All this makes her sound like a monster, but in fact she was very sweet most of the time. Every evening we would all get into our pyjamas and dressing gowns and sit beneath the huge baroque chandeliers in Curty's drawing room, with books everywhere, and a roaring fire, while Curty read to us. We were allowed to knit as we listened and so I did, but I was quite hopeless at it and produced some very lumpy and shapeless garments in the process. There was a bookshelf by the door that led to the dormitories, and on it there always seemed to be a packet of chocolate digestive biscuits. Several of us got into the habit of surreptitiously removing a biscuit on the way to bed. We felt rather wicked but very happy to be able to do this. I can't now imagine that Curty was unaware that this was happening, but perhaps she rather enjoyed the thought of us thinking we were pulling the wool over her eyes.

The worst example of Curty's injustice was the way she chose girls to come with her on her fairly frequent trips to Brighton. There was no fairness in the selection process, no taking turns. Some girls were chosen all the time, others never. I was chosen quite often, at least during my favoured period. What happened was this. You would be sitting in the classroom in the middle of a lesson and the door would suddenly open. Curty would come in and stand there swaying, twisting her beads while she looked silently at the class. Then she would say: 'You, you and you – go to the kitchen and get some sandwiches – I'm taking you to Brighton'. So you would put your work in your desk, go and get the sandwiches (always made with mixed fruit jam out of a very large tin) and you would stand by the gate until Curty came by in her big black car and picked you up. When you got to Brighton you could do what you liked. We usually just wandered the streets looking in shop windows. If anyone had any money we might have a cup of tea and a bun, and once we managed to see a film with James Dean in it. Then at some prearranged time we would meet Curty and drive back to Langford.

One time I was standing at the gate with three or four other girls waiting for Curty to pick us up. We had our jam sandwiches and were looking forward to a day out. We heard the car crunching and roaring on the gravel and we stepped forward expectantly, but Curty drove straight past us and on to the Brighton road, waving cheerily at us as she did so.

Sometimes we were all taken out for special occasions. Once a small group of us ended up visiting an old man who turned out to be Leonard Woolf and who gave us tea on his rolling green lawn and was very gentle and polite with us all. I had been made to read *To the Lighthouse*, which I had found incomprehensible and fascinating at the same time, and was wondering all through the tea whether Virginia had drowned herself in the very river which I suspected flowed down the side of the garden, and if so whether he could sit there every day without thinking about it. And often in the summer we were taken to Glyndebourne to see the operas. There we would sit on the grass with our mixed jam sandwiches, surrounded by people in evening dress with chicken and champagne picnics, and we would get to hear Mozart, which pleased me a lot.

Perhaps partly as a result of my unhappiness, I became very religious at Langford Grove. However, established religion did not really do the trick as far as I was concerned. We used to be taken to church every Sunday, a long walk through rather dreary lanes, but there was something dry and empty about the services, which did not fulfil my need for profound, mystical experiences. Even so I decided to be confirmed, which rather shocked my father, a declared atheist. My mother said she was an agnostic but I think secretly she was rather a believer herself ('I just don't know, darling', she would say if pressed, but she had certainly seemed to like saying prayers with me when I was little). I enjoyed the confirmation classes because I loved the language of the prayer book: 'What is your name?' 'N or M'. For the great day itself I was supposed to have a white dress but in fact Sophie had me made a cream silk one which looked a bit out of place among all the snow whites and which made me look extremely fat. She came to the service, but George did not. In fact I don't think he ever visited me at school. He was withdrawing more and more from our lives, quietly but definitively.

If I was disappointed in Christianity as it was practised in the Protestant church, I found other ways of getting my quota of spirituality. I did this by going for long, solitary walks in the countryside. As I walked I would just put my attention gently on the trees and grass and plants and I would feel as if I saw God in all of them. To pick a leaf seemed liked sacrilege because it was picking a part of God. I was completely in love with nature. I walked a lot, summer and winter, full of powerful, unnameable feelings. I could be swept off my feet by a beautiful sight — there was a copper beech tree on the lawn which, on late summer afternoons, would have its trunk and underside of its leaves suddenly illuminated by the setting sun so that it turned red gold. I used to think it made the place look like heaven. This kind of thing made life at school bearable for me.

Being used to George not being around all that much anyway, I didn't really miss him while I was at school. Missing my mother was the worst thing, but she did write to me a good deal, and about once a month she would come and take me out. Much as I loved seeing her, I had by this time developed a typically teenage sense of embarrassment about her. She was not like the other mothers, who all wore hats and dresses: Sophie always turned up in trousers and a donkey jacket. She was older than the other mothers, too, something I had never noticed when I was little but which I did notice at Langford and which made me feel bad. I never knew exactly how old she was but I could see she was not a young woman. She was still pretty, and she smelled lovely, always of a scent she loved called Marcel Rochas' *Femme*, and she was soft and gentle to hug. But she was worried about looking old and she used to wear a lot of make-up on her face to try and cover up the wrinkles. It was called Max Factor Pancake, and had to be put it on with a little damp sponge. She would wear this, and some lipstick, even when she was in bed at night. I think she could not bear to see her own ageing face at any time.

The days she came to take me out were a lot of fun. Even though she was so obviously sad these days she never lost her ability to enjoy herself, and she always kept her sense of humour. When she came to take me out for a day we would always go to Brighton and we would always have lunch somewhere like Lyons Corner House because we loved the sort of food you got there: baked beans on toast with a poached egg on top, and several cups of very strong tea. She loved tea and would drink it absolutely scalding hot, hiccuping as she sipped from the shock of it. We also enjoyed going out to tea in the sort of tea-shops you could find in lovely old villages, tea-shops with lots of home-made cakes in them. Then we would have what she called a blow-out, which meant eating so much you felt you would never be able to move afterwards. Then after tea she would light up a cigarette. She smoked a lot, far too much, and by the time I was about thirteen she would get me to light her cigarettes as she drove the car. This made me start to enjoy smoking, and soon Cathy and I were buying cigarettes for ourselves and smoking them as we sat at either end of the bath at Lower Mall.

When I was not much more than thirteen she decided to teach me to drive. We used to have lessons on quiet country roads, and I learned fairly quickly how to change gear and get the car to go forward. But something rather unfortunate happened as a result. This was one summer holiday, soon after I had gone to Langford. Our holidays by now consisted of just the two of us, George being occupied elsewhere. We were on our way to visit on old friend of hers, who she always referred to as Morna Haggard: she had been married to Stephen Haggard, an actor who had died in the war. She and her second husband, Richard Elmhurst, lived on a farm at Dollar, in Scotland, with a large family of children including two Haggard boys, Piers and Mark. Sophie and I were going to stay there for a week or so and then go on to Ireland. I had never been to either place before and I was very excited.

It was a long drive to Scotland, up the A1, and you had to stop for the night on the way. So to while away the time, she suggested I might like to drive for a bit, and I took over the wheel. Sophie was tired and soon she started to doze in the passenger seat. Then I saw that we were coming into Doncaster, which I could see was a large town. I had never driven in a town and I started feeling rather nervous. But before I could wake her up and ask her what to do, we had come up to a set of traffic lights and all the cars in front were stopping and I suddenly realised I didn't know how to stop that quickly. I made the effort, but it was not very successful and I crunched straight into the back of another car.

Sophie woke up at once, and said, 'Quickly, quickly, change places!'. But the man in the car in front had seen what was happening and that I was under age. The cars were not much damaged —ours had a dented radiator and his a dented bumper. He told us he was a mechanic, and he said, 'I don't think you want the police called, do you?'. Then he took us back to his garage and he made us pay £20 although his bumper would not cost anything like that much to fix, just so he would not call the police. Sophie was furious and I felt sick and shaky but there was nothing we could do. So we went off to a pub and she bought two gin and oranges, one for her and one for me.

This holiday seems to have been jinxed by some accident-causing demon. The rest of the journey went OK, and we were warmly received by the family. My mother loved Morna, who had lived for a while as a close neighbour during the war. She especially admired her ability to give birth so quickly and easily and with such obvious pleasure. As for me, I was full of admiration for the two handsome blond boys. Mark, who was always called Tiger, was my age and thus rather too young to interest me except as a friend, but Piers was gorgeous and at least seventeen. The best thing about him was that he had his own motorbike. Seeing me gazing at it longingly one day soon after we arrived, he asked me if I would like to have a ride. I said yes. He had to go into town to pick up a prescription for his mother, and would take me along if I wanted, which I did. So off we went, whizzing down the little Scottish roads, the wind in our faces — a thrill I would always enjoy.

When we got to the doctor, Piers carefully parked his bike outside and left me sitting on the back while he ran up the steps to get the prescription. But as he disappeared through the door the bike slowly tipped over sideways, taking me with it, and before I knew where I was I was on the pavement with the bike lying on top of my leg. I yelled, and everyone came rushing out to rescue me. All I felt at first was extreme shock — my leg was black with oil from the exhaust, which had fallen directly on top of it. But by the time we got back to the farm it had started to hurt really badly and a huge blister had come up all over my calf.

So that was the end of any plans we had for going to Ireland. I was laid up for ten days on the sofa, listening to Mark's collection of Lonnie Donegan and Elvis Presley records, the same three or four over and over again. I would never again be able to hear The Rock-Island Line or to anything by Elvis without thinking of that farmhouse living room, full of dogs and small children. When my leg finally healed there was a strange mottled look about it which took many years to disappear.

Of course I got home from school during the holidays, but at first I used to be allowed to travel up to London to go to first nights at the Court as well. I started at Langford in the autumn of the year that the English Stage Company began, and for the whole of the first term I was popping up and down regularly so that I didn't feel left out of what was going on at the theatre. But by the following spring my parents decided that enough was enough and that it was unsettling for me to do this. So I was told I had to give it up. Unfortunately this happened just as a production was about to open that I desperately wanted to see. This was Ionesco's *The Chairs*. I knew Ionesco because he and Mme Ionesco, two tiny French-speaking Rumanians, used to come and have dinner at Lower Mall. Not only that but my father was to play the Old Man and Joan Plowright, who I knew really well too, the Old Woman. The designer was Jocelyn – her first production, in fact. It was an event not to be missed, but I was being told I must miss it.

I simply decided that I was going to participate whether anyone wanted me to or not. I didn't see why I should be left out of an occasion I had always been part of before. So I decided to run away from school. This seemed to me to be a perfectly rational and sensible decision and I made it quite coolly. There was a railway station about half a mile away and I made sure I knew what time the London train stopped there. Then on the day of the first night I simply walked quietly out of the school at break-time, down the drive and out onto the road. I walked purposefully, so that I looked as if I was meant to be there. But inside my heart was pounding like a steam-hammer. With confidence and self-possession I walked up to the railway station, onto the platform. No one saw me, no one stopped me. The train came in and soon I was on it, wild with elation — I had escaped!

I bought my ticket on the train and settled down in the corner, unable to prevent myself from smiling hugely with triumphant delight at my cool cleverness — the plan had worked. Once the train arrived at Victoria I headed for a phone. My mother was at home, getting ready to go to the theatre. 'I'm at Victoria', I told her, 'I've run away from school'.

How did I expect her to react? I don't think I had thought that far. My mother was almost never angry and she was not angry now, but I could tell from her voice that she was very very upset. My triumph was immediately deflated, needless to say, and my cleverness seemed a good deal less clever. She seemed at a loss to know what to say or do, how to react. But she said that since I was there I might as well come and meet her at Sloane Square and she would deal with what to do after the play.

Why did I never stop to think how she would feel? I just didn't think like that. I was determined to do what I wanted and I was also quite used to having my own way. So the sad reaction — a deep deep sadness — was worse by far than any reproaches or anger. But here I was. So we went to the café round the corner from the theatre and had a sandwich and decided I would have to stay the night and go back to school in the morning: she had rung them to say where I was, but could not speak to Curty because Curty had gone off somewhere for the day, no-one knew where.

At last it was time to go to the play. Crowds were standing around on the pavement, pushing their way up the steps of the theatre. I joined them, looking for friendly familiar faces — half the fun of first nights was seeing old friends. But then I saw a face that was less friendly though only too familiar — a face topped with a rakish velvet cloche hat, eyes goitreishly bulging, a neck clinking with beads. Yes, it was Curty. We saw each other at exactly the same minute, the crowds having jostled us into close proximity. A dreadful moment — what would she say?

Curty was quite wonderful. She greeted me with a beaming smile. 'Why didn't you tell me you were coming? We could have travelled up together'. I

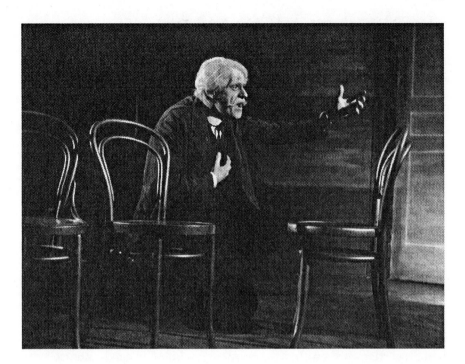

*George in* The Chairs

mumbled a reply — what could possibly be an adequate response to such a question? My mother, as surprised as I was, was pleased to have a chance to talk to Curty, and the two of them disappeared together at the first interval. I did see the play, and it was wonderful. I was sorry by now to have had to have achieved it by these means, which had come to feel shabby and had hurt my mother rather inexplicably more than I could have anticipated. It must have been an agonising evening for her, being the first production Jocelyn had designed, though I did not think of this at the time. But I was not sorry to have been in on such a great event. It was one of my father's huge acting successes, and he looked so adorable in it, a little old Frenchman with a moustache, just the sort of character he felt most comfortable with I believe. The play, which is about two old people filling a room with chairs and ushering in invisible people to sit in them ('Who are all these people, my pet?') was sad and funny and disturbing all at the same time, and it would stay in my mind forever.

Afterwards was going to be the usual first night party and I had been looking forward to being there but now I was not going to be allowed to join in the fun. I never even saw George after the show, though I had been looking forward to that very much – it would have interesting to see how he had reacted to my surprise appearance. But Curty was travelling back to Sussex on the last train and she was going to take me with her. So instead of sipping wine on the stage it was a taxi to Victoria and into a carriage with my headmistress. I expected that now there would be some anger, some reproaches at least from Curty, but they did not materialise. She was kindness itself. She bought me a sandwich and a cup of tea, and we talked little. She told me she would see me next day when we were less tired, and, back at school, I crept into my dormitory and into my cold bed.

In the morning, full of trepidation, I presented myself at Curty's door. Now surely I would be told off or punished. Instead, though, I got a kind, understanding talk. My mother had told Curty that she and my father were breaking up and that I was probably disturbed as a result. The assumption was that this was the reason I had run away. So no more would be said about it, no punishment, no recriminations. In fact Curty and all the teachers were much nicer to me afterwards, more gentle, kind and considerate. This made me feel a great deal worse. As far as I could tell, running away had had nothing to do with the marriage break-up. I just felt like going to see the play so I went. Headstrong, determinedly independent, with little respect for authority, I had simply been putting into practise the principles I had shocked my class with, demonstrating that no-one can be controlled by teachers if they do not want to be.

However, somehow or other the kindness and consideration with which I was treated afterwards did have its effect. It made me feel guilty and it made me think. I did love my mother hugely though I was often irritable and grumpy with her, and it was not a pleasant experience to see how much I had hurt her. This would not be the last time I would upset her: I would go on doing so blithely as long as she lived. But something had happened, some process of thinking about consequences, which slowly, over a long time, would result in my becoming marginally more thoughtful, marginally more aware of the feelings of others. Not much though, and certainly not overnight.

# 8

You might think that my father's slow retreat from my mother, from Lower Mall, and by extension from me, would have made a big difference to my life. In fact it was less traumatic than it might have been. Although it must have prolonged my mother's agony, I think it did have the effect as far as I was concerned of getting me slowly accustomed to his frequent absences. More than anything, though, I was used to his not being there a great deal anyway. He had never been the sort of father who went to work at nine and came home at five: his schedule for most of my life was to disappear after breakfast and not reappear until after the evening performance. There had been times when he was around a bit more, but even when he started to leave he made a point of being at home with us at weekends. Was this because he didn't have the courage to dump my mother overnight even though he really wanted to? This is the interpretation most people have put on it and perhaps it is right. I certainly accepted it as an explanation myself for most of my life. It is only since reading his letters to her, especially the ones he wrote during the war, so full of tenderness and passion, that I have started to wonder whether there was still a part of him that loved and depended on Sophie and found it hard to relinquish her entirely.

So life at Lower Mall went on. Sometimes we would still all go out as a family, as we did when my father was awarded his CBE. We all drove to Buckingham Palace in a hired car, and though we giggled a lot it was impossible not to feel rather overawed by the fact that we were driving through those famous gates and were actually going to see what was inside. In fact the whole thing was a huge anti-climax as we really saw very little. My father was whisked off in one direction and Sophie and I were ushered down a very long and unexciting corridor with a carpet so thick it absorbed all sound of footfalls. We ended up in a huge and cavernous room, empty apart from rows and rows of little gilt chairs facing one end where there was a throne. Along one side was a sort of minstrels' gallery and in it there were minstrels of a sort, playing rather tinkly, palm-court kind of music. Sophie whispered to me that it was a bit like Lyons Corner House.

Then the Queen appeared. We were too far away to see her very clearly but we could see that she was dressed up to the nines, as my mother would say, in heavy oyster satin studded with diamanté, so that she twinkled all

100

over like a fairy. The ceremony began, and it went on and on. As it worked were rather a long way down the pile. But at last it was my father's turn, and there he was looking suitably grave and solemn, kneeling before his sovereign with who knows what revolutionary thoughts in his mind, and having a rather Ruritanian-looking medal put round his neck. At last it was all over and we escaped into our hired car and laughed hysterically. In the evening there was a party on the stage and George insisted that I wore the CBE round my neck all evening: 'The Queen has touched this', he kept saying with mock awe.

Then there were the dinner parties, mostly for the writers. Sometimes these were visiting celebrities, people like Samuel Beckett and Eugene Ionesco, but more often they were the British variety: Arnold Wesker, John Arden and his wife Margaretta D'Arcy, John Osborne, Ann Jellicoe, Doris Lessing, and many others.

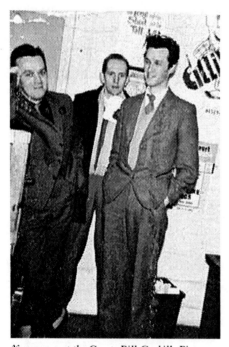

*Young men at the Court: Bill Gaskill, Pieter Rogers and Donald Howarth*

I liked the writers, and some of the assistant directors – Bill Gaskill in particular became an early and lifelong friend – and I enjoyed listening to the conversations about theatre, and art, and life, though I would never dare to say a word. My father sometimes told his dreadful, often-repeated jokes, like the one about the nervous young actor who can't get his one and only line right:

*Actor Manager: Why d'you have to say 'yes-ter-day'? Why can't you just say 'yesterday'?*

*Nervous Young Actor: Just purely narves!*

*Actor Manager: Just purely narves? Then BOO!!!*

Sometimes he also made us play ghastly games: 'If your mother and I were drowning in a river and you could only save one of us, which one would you save?' was one (quite unanswerable), and the other (a sign that I was being treated more like an adult) was 'If you had to sleep with either x or y, which one would you sleep with?' — x or y being the two most repellent people you could think of.

Sometimes the writers asked us to visit them. We spent one rather uncomfortable evening at the Weskers' council flat in Clapton — uncomfortable because, as Arnold has written in his autobiography, he thought my father was patronising them. I'm sure that this was not true, but there was a rather difficult atmosphere all evening. I liked the Weskers a lot — Arnold with his astonishingly bright brown eyes, Dusty big and comfortable and soft seeming (though probably rather tougher on the inside), and, in a corner, Arnold's tiny little mother, dark and twinkly like her son. I think one problem was that no one as staunchly socialist as Arnold could really feel totally at home with George, whose politics were rather more nebulous. He always voted Labour, but he was not a man of rigid beliefs, and I think this irritated card-carrying Leftists like Arnold and Lindsay Anderson. Lindsay told Irving Wardle a story of George asking 'What is a socialist? Am I a socialist?'. For Lindsay this was an illustration of his political confusion, but for me it shows George at his best. I can really identify with that refusal to accept any system wholesale. He wanted to question, to dig deeper, and was unhappy with rigid and dogmatic labelling.

The writer my father liked best was Nigel Dennis, who wrote *Cards of Identity*, *The Making of Moo*, and, in the early sixties, the disastrous *August for the People*. He lived in a big house in the country and we spent several happy Sundays there sitting on the lawn, George and Nigel talking about anything but the theatre. One thing my father especially enjoyed hearing about was Nigel's gardener. A fanatical fan of *The Archers*, this individual was unable to take on board the fact that the characters were played by actors, however much Nigel tried to convince him . One day, Nigel told us, he was hugely relieved when the gardener said to him, 'That new Walter Gabriel is not as good as the old one!'. 'Why not?', asked Nigel, expecting some profound comment on the man's acting abilities. 'The old one would never have planted turnips before February!'

As Tony Richardson and John Osborne became increasingly successful, as they did after starting Woodfall films, we sometimes socialised with them too. I will never forget one miserable evening at John's little house in Woodfall street, sitting on the sofa next to his exquisite wife Mary Ure. She was probably about my height but there was a great deal less of her, and I felt like an elephant sitting next to a fawn. At around this time we also had some hilarious evenings at Lowndes Cottage in Belgravia where the film producer Harry Salzmann was living. Tony and John were doing business with him and he loved to throw parties. Larry Olivier would often be there, and Joan Plowright with whom he was in love but who had not yet parted from her husband. One evening I was overawed to meet Burt Lancaster and Kirk Douglas. There would be masses to eat and masses to drink, and everyone would become extremely jolly.

After Mary Ure's departure John took up with a high-class courtesan called Francine, who was quite the most glamorous person I had ever met. Tall and dark, dripping with ill-gotten diamonds, she was definitely from another world. One evening after some show or party I watched her get into John's large and flashy car. She slid into the driving seat and as he placed himself beside her she tucked up her silk skirt so that the whole extent of her amazingly long, brown, exquisitely shaped legs was visible. Something about the panache of that gesture made a huge impression on me.

One thing that did come to an end after my father left was the family holidays. We still took holidays but it was just me and my mother, unless we could get someone to come with us. When I was about fourteen we had one of the most memorable ones, a trip to the South of France. Sophie took along Claire Jeffries, who had worked as her assistant on various productions, and I took Cathy. My mother had managed to find a house to rent in Gassin, one of the hill-villages overlooking St Tropez.

We had an appalling old car — not the old Austin Seven, which had finally died, but another almost equally inadequate. Again it had no heating and again it had a leaky roof, but we did not worry about this as we were setting out for the warm South. Inside, the window-frames were made of wood, something Cathy and I found very useful. The two of us sat in the back and sang and laughed like maniacs all the way. We were unbelievably silly, but Claire and my mother often laughed with us in spite of their attempts at grown-up gravitas. The thing that made us laugh the most was a game we had devised called 'charming men'. The rules were pretty simple. As you drove through a town or a village, you had to look out of the window and try to catch the eye of a man walking down the street. If you did catch his eye, you gave him a delightful smile, and if he smiled back you shouted 'I've charmed a man!', and made a pencil mark on the window-frame. We were amazingly successful and soon the windows were dark with our little lines. We never tired of this and played it all the way down and all the way back.

When we arrived we had one night in a hotel in St Tropez before making our way up to Gassin. Cathy and I decided to go out and charm some more men. We made our way to the harbour, where there were a great many sailors who we decided were pirates, all dressed rather dashingly in blue and red. Now we discovered that charming men when you are not driving past them in a car is a much more dangerous business. Our smiles were attractive and encouraging and the pirates were certainly attracted and encouraged. But what we had not reckoned with was our close proximity, and soon the pirates were approaching us with hopeful gleams in their black

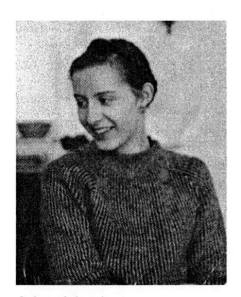

*Cathy aged about sixteen*

eyes. We became nervous and set off rapidly towards the hotel where we took refuge in our room. Looking out at the street below, we could see the pirates lurking about in expectation, presumably, of some further and more frightening form of charm. It took a long time before they realised they were not going to get it and shuffled off back to the harbour. Later, Cathy struck up a friendship with another, less threatening sailor, her Toulon sailor. Having been to school in Paris she talked to him in what she thought was perfect French and was a bit put out that he guessed she was English. I thought him plain and dull, and she was rather hurt that I was not more impressed.

The cottage in Gassin was simple. It was so simple that it did not have any plumbing at all. There was an outside lavatory, but if you wanted to go to the loo at night you had to use a chamber pot. In the morning someone had to empty these over the wall which looked out over a steep hillside with terraced vegetable gardens. These gardens were wonderfully profuse, presumably as a result of all the chamber pots that were emptied over them. The someone who emptied the pots every day was Sophie. I never even thought of doing it. Cathy did, so she told me later, but she couldn't bring herself to and so felt guilty all the holiday. I don't know what Claire thought.

We had a quiet week at Gassin. We went to the beach, and some days we ate a wonderful Provençal soup called *pistou* in the cafe on the terrace. One day we decided to go to Marseilles, but were unable to because a bit fell off the bottom of the car. We went to a garage in St Tropez to get it fixed and some Americans who were hanging around there laughed at the car and asked us if it was held together by sellotape and glue. It was, more or less, but we were very hurt. One night on our way up the hill to Gassin there was a huge thunderstorm and we were all very frightened. To give us courage we sang hymns very loudly, shouting them out against the thunder and lightening and dashing rain. The leaky roof was the least of our problems on that occasion but it did start to matter on the journey back to England. As we drove further and further north, charming men all the way, the weather suddenly turned wet and cold. Sophie stopped in a town and bought us all hot water bottles and plastic macs and we made our way back to England huddled up against the drips. Altogether it had been a great holiday.

Charming men from inside the car was all very well, but what I really wanted was a boy friend. Cathy always seemed to have lots of admirers, and most people at Langford had boys at minor public schools with whom they corresponded fervidly during term-time and exchanged damp kisses in the holidays. But I had no one. This is not to say that I did not have any contact with men, but that was just what they were, men. Men were always kissing me. This all seems rather odd to me now, given my extreme youth and my less than sylph-like figure, but at the time I just took it for granted. It started when I was thirteen — that fateful year when so much seems to have happened. The first person was the son of a friend of Percy's, a hugely tall American in his early twenties by the name of Gene Black. He was not my type, but kind of bullishly good-looking. He came to visit Percy in her studio in Earl's Court Square, and turned up in a most delightful little open-topped sports car which I admired tremendously. Seeing how much I loved it, he invited me to go for a drive, and when we got back to Earls Court Square, instead of getting out of the car at once, he leaned over to the passenger seat and started, much to my astonishment, to kiss me fervently. I was amazed and intrigued, and thought of nothing else for the rest of the day and night. I longed for it to happen again but the next day the opportunity did not arise as we all set off to go out together and travelled in Percy's car. As we made our way out of the studio he managed to fall behind with me, and murmured to me, 'Its a pity we can't go in my car — I won't have a chance to neck with you again'.

*Neck* with you! What was this? Yes, I knew it was an American expression and I had heard it before. But for some reason when he used that word to describe what had happened the day before I started to feel angry and sick. Before he said it I was more than willing to give it another try but now I hated him and hated myself and hated the kisses. And all this had something to do with the word *neck*. I suppose I felt it cheapened the experience. In any case next day he went back to wherever he came from. At least I could now say I had been kissed, even though all I felt was shame and misery about it all.

This was only the first of a series of kisses that from now on seemed to take place quite regularly. Always it was adult men, not boys, and usually on the stage of the Royal Court after a first night. There were always parties, after every first night, and I always went to them, unless I was away at school. Long trestle tables would be put up along one side of the stage and on them would be put bottles and bottles of drinks. I was not very keen on drinking as it made me feel sick and dizzy, but if I had wanted to, no one would have stopped me or even noticed. Everyone else seemed to drink a great deal. The parties went on till very late, so late that my father was able to leave and go to Fleet Street where he could pick up the first editions of the morning papers. These he would bring back to the party and read out the notices of whatever play had just opened. Almost invariably these would be bad notices, outraged and uncomprehending, and he would read them with exaggerated relish, accompanied by cheers and catcalls from the listeners. It was a ritual, and a good one — far better than sitting at home at breakfast, tired and anxious, and having no one but your family to bounce them off against. Here it was the whole theatre family, laughing and roaring and shouting, and that dissipated the depression.

Sometimes I would simply sit in the stalls and watch the party as if it was a continuation of the play. At other times I might be lurking in the wings watching people dancing — a particularly lively party at which there was plenty of this was after the opening of Barry Reckord's West Indian play, *Flesh to a Tiger*. There was Caribbean music and dancing and even limbo dancing which most of us were completely unable to do, and George danced all evening with a Jamaican beauty called Berril Briggs.

It was on these occasions that someone would seize me and start to kiss me: at the *Flesh to a Tiger* party I remember it was a rather unprepossessing black actor, a sad and gloomy sort of chap whose day-job was something to do with London Transport. He did actually try to make a date with me, but usually there was no follow-up to the kissing and the people involved were never very beautiful or memorable. However, it was always interesting, enjoyable and educational. No one ever tried to go further than just kissing and I would not have wanted them to. I knew what the possibilities were as I had read the *Modern Pattern for Marriage*, but for the time being kissing was quite enough. Were these men perverts, child-molesters? I think they must have thought I was much older than I was. Certainly on one occasion when I was rather unpleasantly molested on a dance floor by a very ancient-seeming actor called Hugh Griffiths, from whose lecherous embraces I managed to make a quick escape back to my parents' table, it transpired during the ensuing conversation that he thought I was seventeen rather than the fourteen I actually was. On another occasion I was taken into the bushes in the garden outside the theatre in Stratford by a tall skinny actor and had to be rescued from his passionate clasp by Percy, who had noticed I was missing from the party.

My time at Langford, meanwhile, was coming to an end. I took four O-levels when I was just coming up to fifteen and two (one of them the ill fated maths) just after my fifteenth birthday. The school expected me to stay on and take A-levels there but I was bored and fed up. I played along for a term, read the set books, but as usual did absolutely no work and found, to my horror, that the end of term exams demanded rather more than a cursory reading of the texts. Dismal failures in both English and French — my favourite subjects — decided me, and after rather tearful interviews with both my parents I managed to persuade them to let me leave. Thinking back, it might have been more judicious of them to put their feet down and make me stay on, and I am not even sure if it was legal for me to leave before I was sixteen, but leave I did. Probably their emotional traumas were leaving them with too little energy to fight back.

The problem then was what on earth they were going to do with me now. I wanted to act but was far too young to go to drama school. I quite fancied doing some art, and there was talk of getting me in to the Chelsea Art School but there wasn't enough time to set it up straight away. So it was decided somehow or other that it might be good for me to spend some time in Rome. I could learn Italian and probably find some art classes to go to as well. No-one actually enquired ahead to see if this was really feasible or not: it was just assumed that I would sort it out when I got there. I was fifteen and a half — rather too young, some might think, to be left pretty much to my own devices in Rome, but my parents seemed to believe I would be all right, and all in all I was. I had to have somewhere to stay, and George for once involved himself in the process of sorting this out. He contacted some people at the British Council who found me a place with a couple of ladies who had a flat near the Borghese Gardens. I didn't know a word of Italian, so I went for some weeks to Italian lessons with Teresa Collingwood's half-brother's Italian wife Vera, who taught me the basics: *Mi chiama Harriet — sonno Ingelsa'* and so on. Then it was time to go.

My need to get to Italy coincided with George's need to have a holiday. In fact he seemed to be on the verge of some kind of breakdown, presumably a result of the strain of the break-up and the Jocelyn business, but being a pretty self-absorbed teenager I didn't give this much thought. So he decided to go to Italy himself, and off we set in his old Alvis car, the one with the long shiny black bonnet and the lamps like two large blue eyes on the front. The car caused a sensation as we made our way south through France and into Italy: people used to gather round it and stare. It was the usual George kind of journey — the *Guide Michelin*, the little family-run hotels — but the first and only one we ever made alone. So it was a very special time for me and I remember it as a really happy few days, even though George did not talk much — he clearly had a lot on his mind. He did, however, tell me the names of things as we drove through France, and sometimes he learned them himself for the first time. One he particularly liked was the name of the belisha beacon: *le clignotant* (the blinker, the winker, the flasher). Every time we came to a level crossing we said the name together: *passage à niveau*.

On our first stop, as we walked down the street, he took a look at my shoes. They were completely disreputable — flat ballet-type shoes, but absolutely falling apart, with holes in the uppers and the soles falling off. 'Are they the only ones you have?'. They were (God knows what my mother was thinking of) and I was fond of them. 'Well, they look rather awful'. So we bought another pair.

After dinner on our second night, in some small town or other, we caught sight of a poster advertising a performance that night by a small travelling theatre company, and decided to go. It was absolutely terrible but extraordinarily enjoyable. There was an ageing leading lady, dressed entirely in the brightest imaginable pink satin and covered in thick orange make-up. She was being courted by a very plump gentleman whose face was also bright orange. There were sword fights, tears and laughter, deaths and reconciliations. It was one of the few plays I ever saw with my father at which he did not walk out before the end.

One night we stayed at a place that was probably the nicest hotel in the world. I have spent the rest of my life wondering where it was and if it still exists. It was in the middle of a huge forest and rather difficult to find. When we did finally arrive, we found a small *manoir*, run by a family and still furnished as if it was their own home. There were old beds, old china, old dressers, old wardrobes, all beautiful but all falling apart, rather like my discarded shoes. We were almost the only guests. The dinner was quietly wonderful — soup in a huge tureen, a simple but delicious main course, and for dessert — pears. Not just any old pears — both George and I agreed that they were without any doubt the best pears we had ever eaten.

At last we arrived in Rome, and found our way to the flat where I would be spending the next few months. Meeting the family was a bit of a shock. They were not quite what we had had in mind. The two I would be living with were a couple of ladies well into their sixties, a widow and her spinster sister. They spoke not a word of English. The widow had a son, a policeman, who did speak English but he lived somewhere else. Well, I was supposed to be learning Italian, and this would certainly do it. In the evening George and I went to a reception at the British Embassy, where we stood beneath twinkling chandeliers eating canapés and drinking champagne. The next day he left for the coast, off to lick his wounds. He was a little worried about leaving me, I could tell, but he did his best to look cheerful and optimistic. And so began my strange Italian visit.

The first question to be answered was what was I to do with myself? The old ladies did not know and nor did I. After my father left the old spinster sister took me for a walk round the neighbourhood. She walked very slowly and every now and then she stopped, coughed, and spat on the pavement, hiding her mouth discreetly behind her hand as she did so. I had never seen anyone do that before, and it made me realise I had landed in an alien culture. I certainly felt rather strange at first, homesick and disoriented. One compensation was that the food was brilliant. Our main meal was lunch and lunch started with pasta, but pasta far more delicious than any I had ever tasted before. Then we had meat and vegetables, and fruit. In the evening it was pasta again, but the thing I liked best was that if we had had spinach at lunch it reappeared cold in the evening and we ate it with olive oil, lemon, salt and black pepper. Simple but wonderful. So the meals were a highlight, but I had to find something to do for the rest of the day.

My Italian improved very rapidly — it had to. I learned to use the buses and every day I went into the city or to the Borghese Gardens. I walked and walked. Soon I knew Rome like the back of my hand, or kept thinking I did, until I rounded some corner or dived into some alley and found somewhere new and even more beautiful. I spent hours in museums and even more hours in churches, which I loved so much more than the cold grey Protestant churches in England. I would cross myself with the holy water and breathe in the incense and wish I had been born a Catholic.

The art lessons proved to be a non-starter. I managed to discover where the main art-schools were but I was either too frightened to go in or if I did, people looked at me as if I was a little crazy. So it was up and down the Spanish steps, in and out of churches, endless window-shopping, coffees in cafes round the Roman ruins. There was a constant undercurrent of fending off men who winked and pinched but were almost certainly quite happy to be fended off.

Then suddenly, in the middle of this rather lonely but very enjoyable time came a quite different sort of interlude. This was the arrival of a film company making a film called *The Nun's Story*. The star of the film was Audrey Hepburn, who I admired more than anyone in the world — if only I could look like her. Alas I never managed to meet her, though I did see her once at a distance. Also in the film was Peggy Ashcroft, who had brought Eliza and Nicky out with her. Another actress who was there was someone I knew because she had been in plays at the Court. Her name was Rosalie Crutchley, but she was always, for some unknown reason, called Bun. I thought her breathtakingly beautiful, very Spanish looking, with long straight black hair and a dark, fine-boned face. Her voice seemed very comforting, deep and strong, and above all I found her wonderfully funny.

Peggy was rather occupied with filming, but once she managed a day off and the company gave her a car with a chauffeur who took us all out for a trip to the Appian Way. The car was extremely grand and had electric windows, the first any of us had ever seen, and we all played with them all the way. When we arrived at the Appian Way, which is all lined with ancient tombs, Peggy asked the chauffeur to let us out to walk and look at them, and so he did. But after we had been walking for a few minutes we became aware of a quiet purring sound behind us and, looking round, discovered that the chauffeur was following us down the road, keeping at a discreet distance, a fact that was funny but rather disconcerting.

Later that same evening we ended up at a restaurant which was perched among olive trees on a terraced hillside. We sat outside under the vines and ate deliciously. The waiter was very proud of his English, which was rather formal and obsequious, so we decided to play a rather silly joke on him. When it was time to pay, we called him over, and Bun, in her grandest voice, said, 'Could we have the William, please?'. The hope was that he would think this was how the truly posh in England asked for the bill. He looked rather surprised, but hurried off to fetch it. Unfortunately by the time he got back we were all in hysterics, which rather dented the impression we were trying to give.

I saw a little of Eliza and Nicky that week, but I saw most of Bun. She seemed only too happy to go out of her way to spend time with me, and took me out several times. Perhaps she felt sorry for me, but I hope she enjoyed it too. I certainly did, as we seemed to share a sense of humour and spent a lot of our time laughing. One day she took me to a famous garden just outside Rome. We found it deeply disappointing. It was all divided into little brown terraces running up the side of the hill and we walked gloomily down wondering what all the fuss was about. Then, as we reached the bottom, we looked up, and at that moment someone turned on a tap and the whole place was transformed. Every terrace had fountains, and the water shot up in sparkling jets, up high into the air. It was breathtakingly magical.

All too soon the film company left, and it was back to street wandering and church visiting. I was completely swept away by the churches — the gold, the statues, the paintings, the lingering incense, the occasional faint sound of chanting. I had not managed to warm to the churches in England in spite of my strong desire for some kind of religious experience, but here in Rome I felt that I understood what churches could and should be like. I did not attempt to go to any services, but I spent a great deal of time wandering around them or just sitting quietly.

The other thing I enjoyed was window-shopping. I developed a desperate desire for a pair of beautiful Italian suede shoes, but I was on a budget (and, amazingly, managing to stick to it) and found nothing that I could afford. Then one day, on my wanderings, I found a little shop in a side street where the shoes were half the price of any I had seen. I tried some on and they were heaven — soft suede, like a glove on your foot, with little heels and pointed toes. So I bought them and transported them home, and though I rarely wore them I had the immense pleasure for the first of many times in my life of finding something truly lovely at a bargain price.

I suppose I was in Rome for about six or eight weeks, but in some ways it seemed a lot longer. My Italian got rather good, and by the end I was certainly thinking in the language. Above all what I gained from it was independence. Afterwards I would never fear going to strange places or being by myself, and in fact to this day I deliberately seek opportunities to wander aimlessly in strange foreign towns and feel trapped by having to spend too much time with others on holidays.

I wonder now how Sophie was, left alone at home while I was at school or in Rome, and my father holidaying or spending increasing amounts of time with Jocelyn. Certainly she must have been pretty desperate, lonely and miserable. It is almost inconceivable, though, sadly, only too true, that I did not think about this at the time. It was around this time that she took on a live-in housekeeper: someone to help with the housework, obviously, but also perhaps for a bit of company. To say this plan was not a success hardly encompasses the awfulness of the results. The person she employed was called Hilda Ormsby. She was a dumpy little woman on the wrong side of middle age. She always wore a drooping tweed skirt and one of a selection of faded, felted beige-coloured jumpers and, to our amused horror, appeared to have a third breast situated above and between the other two rather pendulous ones. Cathy and I said that she was a witch, as they were reputed to have three breasts, or nipples anyway. But this bulge must, I think, have been a handkerchief, something she was greatly in need of as she spent a lot of her time crying. In fact she hardly did any work at all, and this in itself added to my mother's burdens. Worse still, every evening she would come into the sitting room where Sophie was trying to work or to relax, fling herself onto the sofa, and burst into tears. Many hours of my mother's time were spent trying, uselessly, to comfort her, and it took several months before she could be persuaded to move out of our house. After this it was back to cleaning ladies, one of whom, Mrs Pickett, used to bring her tiny son to work with her. We were much amused, and amazed, to learn that she had gone through nine months not knowing she was pregnant and had given birth to this, her second child, in the lavatory. Unhappy though she was, Sophie could always be made to laugh, and this was the sort of thing she really enjoyed hearing about.

# 9

George, despite his problems and his increasing absence, was still my father, but he was also the father of the Royal Court (with Tony as his rather Oedipal son), and the father-figure of the writers and the assistant artistic directors. So these people had to be nurtured and educated and encouraged too. Part of this process was the Writers' Group, which Bill Gaskill started running when I was about fifteen. The intention of this was to let the writers get together and work on improvisation: it was an opportunity to see how something might work in practice that they were trying to get right on the page. Bill and I had always got on well, and he invited me to go along and join in. Of course I went like a shot – I always wanted to join in and belong. The meetings were held at the house of one of the writers, Ann Piper, and luckily she lived just two doors away from us at number 7 Lower Mall, though her house was much bigger than ours. We would meet in her huge living room, on the first floor, overlooking the river. There were usually about ten people there: Arnold Wesker, Ann Jellicoe, Donald Howarth, Edward Bond, Keith Johnstone, others I've forgotten. Keith became something of a friend and indeed I had a rather strange and awkward episode with him a few years later. I always found him fascinating: big and bony, odd and interesting. Wherever he went he carried all his belongings, mostly papers, in large carrier bags, and frequently had also bags of raw vegetables like peas which he was constantly popping out of their pods into his mouth. I liked the way his mind worked: it was not like anyone else's. I've never forgotten a Christmas card he sent which he had drawn himself. It showed a reindeer with a small boy curled up in its stomach. The boy's mother was standing nearby in a doorway, and the caption said: 'Come in out of the reindeer'. Keith and Ann Jellicoe were living together in a flat in Holland Park which was all painted white with chairs hung on hooks on the wall, just like the flat Ann would write into her play *The Knack.*. They had a lodger, the photographer Roger Mayne, who was incredibly shy but had one of the sweetest smiles you could imagine. A bit later he and Ann would get married.

One of the first Writers' Group meetings I went to was a disaster as far as I was concerned. Keith Johnstone was working on a play about a giant and the improvisation exercise was simple: just imagine you are a giant and describe what you can see. For some reason I had to go first. I stood up in front of the group, devoid of ideas and feeling desperately self-conscious. Seeing the river and the lights outside the window, I tried to imagine myself a little bigger, a lot taller, and I described London spread beneath my feet, the streets, the houses, all looking tiny. I did my best but I felt amazingly dull and lacking in ideas. After I had finished I sat down and others followed me in the exercise. Their giants were so much bigger than mine! They didn't just see a tiny bit of the London landscape, they could see the whole world, the entire universe spread out before them. To me this meant that their minds were so much bigger, so much more creative than mine. I felt that I did not have any imagination, that my thinking was limited, that I didn't have the free play of creativity that everyone else had.

Perhaps I was being a bit unfair on myself. I was after all only fifteen, and here I was standing up in front of a group of lively, radical, experimental writers and expecting to shine. But despite my rather odd education I had yet to learn that it was permissible to blast through the barriers and have fun, in the head, that is. I suppose it was quite brave of me to be going to the Writers' Group at all, and this uncomfortable experience did not stop me from going. Everyone was very nice to me and I enjoyed the social aspect of it all a great deal. I found the writers so interesting. I was very drawn to Edward Bond although he never said a word, and I had no idea what strange political thoughts were in his head. When his plays started to be put on I loved them and often found them terribly funny even though many people were shocked by their blackness: I particularly liked *Early Morning*, which was partly about Queen Victoria being a lesbian (John Brown was a woman, and played by Marianne Faithfull), in which people had their body parts removed and eaten. I laughed till it hurt, though audiences rarely shared my amusement and walked out in their droves.

One day I finally managed to do an improvisation that actually took off. Ann Jellicoe had started writing *The Knack* and had brought along a scene that was not working out. It was all to do with people moving a bed. Bill Gaskill and I stood up to do this, and he quickly started insisted that the object we were moving was not a bed.

*It's a piano!*
*No it's not, it's a bed.*
*It's a piano!*
*It's a bed, a bed, a bed!*

Ann really liked what we did, and the scene ended up in the play more or less verbatim.

One day we had a guest at the group, a writer from Africa called Wole Soyinka. After the meeting there was a party and we all drank quite a lot of wine, even me — I was trying to get to like the experience. At some point Wole and I found ourselves wandering off down the road towards Hammersmith, perhaps just to get a breath of fresh air. He was very sweet and kind to me, putting his arm round my shoulders but not making a pass at me. He told me I was too young and he had too much of a sense of responsibility, which made a change. As we headed down Bridge Avenue towards King Street we encountered a man with whom for some reason we struck up a conversation. He invited us to go and have a drink in his flat and so we did, sitting in his rather sad bedsit among the faded chintz, a hissing gas fire in the grate, sipping warm beer while he and Wole had a rather stilted conversation. Then I was taken home to my front door and sent in with a gentle kiss on the cheek.

Another extremely rowdy party at Ann Piper's took place in the summer. Perhaps by this time I was sixteen. I can still remember what I wore: a lovely dress my mother had made me out of a sort of heavy cotton with a very bold print of brightly coloured flowers. I think this must have been during the phase when she had a job designing clothes for a firm called Berketex. Although still rather chubby I had started to lose a little weight and I thought the dress really suited me. It had a low neck, a tight bodice and a very full skirt. It was at this party that I got really drunk for the first time. I spent most of the party sitting at the kitchen table with Arnold Wesker and some of the other writers. There were bottles and bottles of red wine and we seemed to have discovered a great secret which was that, however drunk you were, at the moment when you took a sip of wine you became for that instant completely sober. We tried this again and again and were delighted with the results.

Soon we decided it was time to inspect the baby. Ann had recently given birth and this tiny child was peacefully sleeping in a cradle in the next room. Arnold persuaded me to go and have a look at her. The room was rather dark and once we were in there he shut the door and started to kiss me. After a while we went reluctantly back to the kitchen and then Michael Geliot, one of the assistant directors, also decided he wanted to go with me to inspect the baby and the same thing happened again. Percy told me quite recently that in her opinion Michael Geliot had been 'mad about' me, but I must say if he was I certainly wasn't aware of it, though perhaps the kissing should have alerted me.

A few weeks later I went on an expedition to Bristol with some of the writers: Arnold, Keith and Ann Jellicoe. We drove down in someone's car, to see a play by a writer who was supposed to be good but which in the end turned out to be totally unmemorable. Afterwards we went out for a meal and drank a great deal again. Then we went for a walk out onto the Clifton Suspension Bridge and I was quite overcome by the height of it, experiencing a strange desire to climb onto the parapet and sail gently down onto the shining mud below. But I did not. It was on this expedition that Arnold told me that he would really like to sleep with me but that he was 'too much of a moral coward'. He explained that this meant he was afraid of what my father would say, and told me that many of the writers felt the same. I was quite pleased about this, as I was definitely not ready to go to bed with anyone. I imagine has was right about George, too.

It was my association with the Writers' Group that got me going on the first Aldermaston March. I was not a particularly political person but even I could see how necessary it was to protest against the bomb. In fact the whole issue loomed very large for me and I was quite anxious about it — I used to wake up in the night and wonder if I would live to be grown up. Everyone was very excited about the march. Most of the writers and

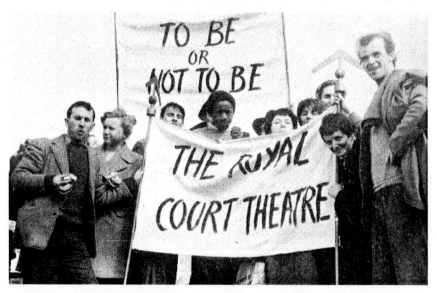

*The Aldermaston March. Arnold Wesker, Dusty Wesker, Peter Gill, Wole Soyinka, Miriam Brickman, Ann Jellicoe, Keith Johnstone, Daphne Hunter, Anthony Page*

directors from the Court were going and my parents, as usual, saw no reason to stop me. Unlike each subsequent year, this march started in London and ended up three days later at Aldermaston in Berkshire. It was a walk of fifty miles. I needed a sleeping bag for the overnight stays and managed to borrow one from Wayland Young, a writer who lived in a rather grand house in Bayswater.

The weather was appalling, dark, cold, and rainy, but morale was incredibly high. Just a few hundred people, cheered on by less hardy souls, set off on the first stretch from London, the Royal Court contingent marching as a group. There was Arnold and Keith, Bill Gaskill, Doris Lessing, Lindsay Anderson — even John Dexter, new to the Court, came along to join in. No one had really suitable footwear and by the time we reached the first overnight stop, a village hall near Slough, all our feet were a mass of blisters. Keith said, as he removed his thick woolly socks, 'Oh look, there's a foot on my blister!'. Someone had brought a darning needle and some white wool, which we all threaded carefully though the blisters where it absorbed the liquid and, hopefully, allowed them to heal overnight. Then we snuggled down in our bags on the hard floor and tried to get some rest.

By the end of the three days, when we reached Aldermaston (numbers by then swollen to perhaps a few thousand) we were all absolutely exhausted, legs aching, feet in shreds. But the sense of elation was incredible. All the way down supporters had been standing by, cheering us on, and providing us with soup and bread along the road. At the head of the march was Bertrand Russell, wiry and white-haired, marching next to the indomitable Jaquetta Hawkes. Behind them a string of groups, people who had travelled from all over the country, each with a banner. Everyone sang, or chanted (the Writers' Group had their own slogan: 'William Shakespeare, William Blake — We are marching for their sake'). I fell in for a while with a group of Young Communists and was briefly swept away by their idealism, singing the Red Flag with the best of them. I took down addresses and details and decided I would join when I got home but in the event I never did. It would be a long time, though, before the excitement of this occasion died away — for weeks afterwards the only people I wanted to be with were those who had shared the experience.

The March became an annual event, though after the first year it went the other way, starting at Aldermaston and ending up at Trafalgar Square where there was a huge rally. No doubt it was better organised, and certainly more people went, but though I joined in every year, no march ever came up, for me, to the excitement and the sense of communal idealism of that first soggy and exhausting weekend.

The reason I was able to join in with so many of the writers' activities at this point in my life was that, after I came back from Rome, I was being educated (after a fashion) in London. I did have one term at the Chelsea Art School, my mother somehow having managed to persuade them to take me on as a part-timer. Essentially what this did was to enable me to see that art, however much I might enjoy it as an activity, was not going to be a career for me. I joined in classes in still life, life drawing and composition and felt completely overawed by the talent of the students. They were all a good three or four years older than I was, but even so I could see that my rather limited abilities were never going to develop to the stage that theirs were at. So at the age of sixteen I decided that perhaps it would be a good idea to take my A-levels after all. I say I decided, as my parents seem to have allowed me to do pretty much whatever I liked.

My old friend Teresa Collingwood was by this time going to school in London, at a very grand place called Queen's College in Harley Street, and it was there I decided I too would like to go. I think it must have been expensive, but this was not advanced as a reason for not going. I never did hear my parents say that we could not afford anything, though my father was earning, relatively speaking, a pittance at the Court and my mother's income was erratic, to say the least. In any case, in September I started at the school, and had quite an enjoyable year there. Catherine was in London at the same time, and she and I used to meet for lunch at one of the big department stores in Oxford Street, or I would hang around with Teresa and some of her friends — one of the good things about Queen's College was that you were treated like a responsible person and allowed out during the lunch hour. I liked the lessons, too, having realised that you did actually have to put something into them. I have no recollection now of what texts we were reading, apart from Milton's *Comus*, which I loved and which I remember participating in a production of at the end of term. So all in all I was getting on quite well, but I had the feeling that things were progressing rather slowly. So halfway through the second term I asked one of the teachers when we were going to sit the exam.

*At the end of next year, of course.*
*Next year?*
*Yes, next year.*
*I thought it was this year!*
*No, next year.*

This was a blow! At Langford, for all its ropy teaching, we had been going to complete the A-level course in a year and I had no idea that this was not common practice. I couldn't hang around doing this for two years, or at least that was how I felt. So once again it was tears, discussions, and an agreement wrung from George and Sophie that I could leave at the end of the school year and do — what? I had decided what I really wanted to do, and that was go to drama school. I'm not sure what George thought of this decision, but at least he helped me to choose a school — LAMDA — because he thought it was the best: many of the teachers there were ex-Old Vic School students. Unfortunately when I did the audition in the summer I was turned down. They said it was on the grounds of my age, as I would have been only just seventeen when the term began, and perhaps this was true. Lyn Redgrave, who was the same age, auditioned at the same time as I did and was turned down also, though in the event she managed to get accepted at the Central School and so did start that year. I however was to take a year out and get some experience in the theatre.

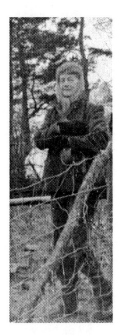

It was while all this was going on that my father finally and irrevocably moved out of Lower Mall. He and Jocelyn set up home together at last, in Rossetti Studios, in Flood Street, Chelsea. There is no doubt that he was very happy there. But for my mother this final move was, I believe, devastating. I think she must have always hoped that his affair with Jocelyn would follow the course of his relationship with Annette in 1939 and would in the end come to a close, leaving him free to come back to her. So when he went, even though he had been with us only at weekends, it was a terrible blow. The downstairs extension, for so long filled with his books, his wooden armchair, his old check dressing-gown hanging on the door, his ties in the wardrobe, his hard plywood bed in the corner, was suddenly empty of anything associated with George and their long relationship — by the time he left they had been together for more than twenty-five years. Had she been another kind of person perhaps she would not have stood for the long drawn out process of his leaving — perhaps she could and would have said, go, just go. But even a tiny shred of hope is enough to stop you doing that and she could not let go of that shred even though she had come to despair and to hate herself and to believe that he hated her. A sad letter he wrote her, undated but certainly from this time, shows what their relations had become:

*Sophie in Wales soon after George moved out*

*Dear Sophie,*
*Although I do not agree with everything you say in your letter, it does not matter as broadly speaking I think it is right and sensible and facing the facts, as you put it. It is never pleasant to compromise, but life seems to be like that.*

*Only one point I want to make. I do not dislike you or find your presence distasteful in any way. It is not that. I will do what I can not to worsen your feeling of tension, which is, naturally, acute at present, because I think it is of paramount importance that you should try to find your way to re-open yourself to the world and give all the things you have to give, which is a very great deal, without condemning yourself to an attitude which will make you feel miserable and useless, and make other people pity you; there is no reason why this should happen but only you can avoid it. I am quite sure of this.*

    *Love,*

        *G.*

I don't think he did dislike her but I am sure it was a huge relief to leave for good. Quite apart from his deep love for Jocelyn and their desire to be together, his guilt and shame at leaving my mother must have been greatly intensified by her reproachful presence — a sad, thin, visibly ageing ghost reminding him of earlier and happier days.

As for me, I think I too was unprepared for the blow of his final departure. You can get used to anything and I had got used to his part-time presence, but when he packed his things and went I did certainly feel what children in that position invariably feel, that it was me he was leaving. My feeling — and this lasted for a very long time — was that he was in some way disappointed in me and that his new family was somehow providing him with pleasures and joys which I had not been able to supply. Because he had not just got Jocelyn, he had inherited an army of stepchildren, or sort-of stepchildren since he and Jocelyn were so resolutely against marriage. My ex-playmates the Lousadas all seemed to be so much more confident and successful than I was: Sandra well on the way to a great career as a photographer, Jenny doing supremely well at art school, the twins so rosy and jolly. They all seemed to be always laughing, though I sometimes wondered if they had quite the same kind of silly fun that we had had at home when I was small. It was hard to imagine George dressing up as a lady, or pretending to club people with a rolled-up newspaper at breakfast, in this household.

Certainly a different side of George was in evidence at Rossetti Studios. In many ways, however, the change obviously did him the world of good. He was now a slender and handsome man, elegantly dressed in clothes from the fashionable new men's shops which were springing up all along the King's Road, and, though clearly stressed and overworked he was just as clearly fulfilled in ways that it would have been churlish to deny him. And, though I felt at times that I had lost him, I never lost him entirely. He still popped in to Lower Mall for Sunday lunch from time to time, and he made a point of regularly taking me out for the evening. Sometimes we

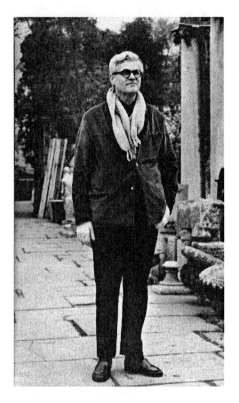

*George newly slender and elegant*

would go and see a film which he would sleep all the way through, sometimes a play, which was a bit of a mixed blessing as he could never bear to stay for more than just the first act. This was not only frustrating, since I never got to find out what happened, but also embarrassing, as the whole cast always knew he was there and we had generally been given complimentary seats. I think it also fine-tuned my own critical sense, and I have noticed with interest that over the years I have become more, rather than less, tolerant of poor performances, especially those in which in some way the hearts of those concerned are in the right place. Sometimes we simply went out for dinner in one of the small French restaurants in Soho that he liked so much. I think it may have been in his favourite, L'Escargot Bienvenu, that the waiters thought (or pretended to think) I was his girl friend, something which seemed to please him a great deal.

Of course, once he and Jocelyn were settled at Rossetti Studios I was able to go and stay there sometimes. Jocelyn must inevitably have found this rather awkward, but she was invariably kind and welcoming, though I still felt rather like a cuckoo in the nest. I was always measuring myself up against the Lousada children, who seemed so happy and successful and good-looking, and finding myself wanting. On one weekend I decided to make some toffee and succeeded in burning it and ruining two saucepans in the process. Everyone was very nice about it, but I felt that in some way it exemplified my clumsiness and stupidity. So although I never entirely lost my father, I never managed to shake off the feeling that I had been rejected for better, brighter, livelier, more creative replacements.

It was in the summer of the year that my father moved out that I had the biggest adventure of all. Not yet seventeen, I went off on my own to spend the summer holidays in North Carolina with a cousin of George

Goetschius. This person was known as Cousin Charles, although his name was not really Charles at all, it was Larry Glenn. How he came to be called Charles by us all (and by himself) is one of the many mysteries about him that I never did clear up. He had turned up on the doorstep of Lower Mall quite unexpectedly the previous autumn and had stayed for many months. He had, unquestionably, swept us all entirely off our feet. I don't think George had even known of his existence, but he was indeed George's cousin, though rather a distant one. Tall, skinny, elegant, gay, with chronic arthritis, which gave him appalling pain from time to time, he was frighteningly charming. He was a poet and a great lover of literature, which he would recite to us endlessly in his delightful Southern drawl — he knew by heart the entire works of Saki and would make us all weep with laughter with his dramatic renditions of these very funny stories ('She was a good cook as good cooks go, and as good cooks go, she went'). One warm spring day he took me rowing on the Serpentine and recited Tennyson to me: 'Dressed in white samite, mystic, wonderful'. Afterwards he wrote me a poem, long since lost, and my heart was given entirely over to adoring him. My mother, who was tender-hearted, loved him too, as indeed everyone who met him did. I never heard him say anything unkind about anyone.

When at last he decided he had to leave, he asked my parents if I could go and spend the summer in the house he shared with his aged great-aunt Edna, in a tiny town called Black Mountain in North Carolina. My mother found the idea distinctly worrying, but my father, to his credit, said that if I wanted to go I should be allowed to go. And want to go I certainly did. So it was that Sophie put me on a boat at Tilbury Docks and, full of misapprehension, waved me off for a two-month stay in America. A huge grey liner, owned by Greeks but run by Germans, the ship called first at Cherbourg where we picked up a large contingent of immigrants from all over Europe who were setting off for a new life in Canada and who spent most of the voyage weeping for their abandoned homes.

The voyage was not a lot of fun. The food was harsh and Germanic, likewise the crew, who seemed to have little sympathy for or interest in the passengers. I was sharing a cabin but the people concerned were so faceless that they have been entirely erased from my memory. As soon as we hit the Atlantic everyone began to be violently seasick, so that it was impossible to go anywhere on deck without finding people vomiting over the side or onto the deck itself. I, for some reason, although I had always been very seasick in small boats, did not succumb to it on this journey, but I did feel rather unwell and developed a badly upset stomach. I went to see the doctor (German) who prescribed me lots of strong tea without milk. I did as I was told but had to force it down as it was absolutely vile — a thick black herbal stew, quite unlike any tea I had ever drunk before.

As the ship was heading for Canada we passed through the north Atlantic and one day everyone rushed out on deck to see huge icebergs drifting slowly past. The sight of them looming up out of the dark could have evoked thoughts of the Titanic (I had been terrified by a film of this a few years earlier and had to be taken weeping from the cinema) but in fact I was not afraid. All I felt at this time was rather numb and quite unable to conceive of what the coming weeks had in store for me. I did not, however, see anything particularly odd in setting off into the blue completely unaccompanied.

As we reached the entrance to the Hudson River, Canada appeared, looking surprisingly dull. The immigrants wept still more at the sight of their new country. The ship docked at Montreal and we all disembarked. No one was there to meet me: that was not the deal. The deal was that I had to find my own way to New York. I had one large case, which somehow appeared on the dock, and I managed to get a taxi to the Greyhound Bus Station. I also, responsibly, managed to send my mother a telegram to say I had arrived safely.

The Greyhound Bus from Montreal to New York City was a journey of about eleven hours, and I dozed a good deal of the way. I remember a lot of shouting at the US border, but I never found out exactly what was going on. At last, late in the night, we arrived at the bus station in New York, which was rather spookily underground. This time I should have been met, but there was no sign of anyone. I began to panic rather — where was Cousin Charles? What should I do? Several large men, bus company officials, noticing that I seemed to be rather lost, kindly came and spoke to me. We established that I believed Cousin Charles had been going to stay with another cousin, Cousin James Golightly. I did not have his address but luckily one of the men managed to find it in the telephone directory.

And so it transpired that Cousin Charles had been delayed, but that he had booked me into a hotel for the night — he would come and collect me in the morning. I have often wondered why he did not attempt to convey this information to the Greyhound Bus Station. A taxi took me to the hotel, which was luxurious, with a huge bed, and a TV with many channels. I slept lightly, aware all night of howling sirens in the streets outside. In the morning my breakfast appeared, toast with coffee and a glass of freshly squeezed orange juice sitting in a bowl of ice, which amazed and enchanted me.

Finally, after breakfast, Cousin Charles appeared. I was extremely glad to see him. He offered no explanation for his absence the day before and I never did find out why he had been delayed. He took me to Cousin James Golightly's smart brownstone house, which was beautifully and lushly furnished with antiques and fine books. We had a most refined lunch, Cousin

James being a most refined person (gay also), but time was passing and soon we had to leave to get another Greyhound Bus which would take us all the way to North Carolina, a journey of some twenty-three hours.

The New York weather had been warm and sticky, but it got warmer and stickier still as we headed south. We passed through Winston Salem and talked about witches (though that was a different Salem) and about cigarettes. On the bus were many black people, and when we stopped at bus stations for rest and food I was extremely shocked to discover that while we were ushered into a large, almost empty, air-conditioned waiting-room, there was just a tiny space for all the black people to cram into. Our side said Whites Only over the door. I had never seen anything like this before and it made me feel deeply uncomfortable.

At last, after a long journey, we arrived in Ashville, North Carolina, and a friend met us and drove us to Cousin Charles's house. Now, however, I had to learn to call him Larry, as that was what everyone here called him. The house was on Montreat Road, Black Mountain, and mountains were indeed everywhere, thickly covered with pine woods. Larry told me there were many bears to be met there. All down the road were large old clapboard houses, each standing alone in its own yard, each with a big veranda on the front. In one of these lived Larry's Aunt Edna. Eighty years old, strong and wiry and bright, she claimed to have brought Larry up, or at least to have cared for him since he was quite young.

The other inhabitant of the house, although I suspected that he actually slept in a shack in the garden, was someone referred to as the nigger. His name was Jim and he was the odd-job man and gardener. Old and grizzled, he had marks on his legs where the chains had been when he was on the chain gang, for what reason I never learned.

My bedroom was at the top of the stairs, with a big window looking out over the street and a large iron bedstead. Larry's room was across the landing. The room where he spent most of his time, though, was his downstairs study, which I admired tremendously. All the walls were painted dark green, there was a large dark leather desk, and books everywhere. I thought it the most grown-up and sophisticated room I had ever seen.

Aunt Edna was very kind to me but seemed always a little remote. Probably she was rather surprised to have me there and wondering why Larry had asked me to stay. If so, she was not alone, as it turned out. Rather surprisingly she did all the cooking herself and I grew quickly to like Southern food — corn bread, which appeared regularly, and okra, which I had never tasted before and which was often cooked with tomatoes.

There seemed to be no clear plan of action for me while I was there. Essentially Larry would take me out and about to visit his friends and

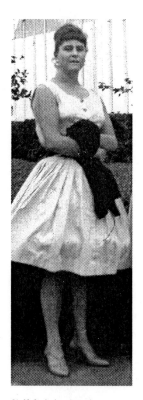

*Jail-bait in America*

relations. His brother Jim lived in a big house not far away with a wife and two small children, and we spent some enjoyable days sitting on the grass and making ice cream in their ice-cream machine. I say machine but this did not have a motor. It was all made from wood, and into it went cream, sugar, and peaches, peeled and chopped. Somewhere else went cracked ice. Then you had to sit there for an unbelievably long time cranking the handle round and round. It was exhausting and your arm ached like mad. You thought the ice cream would never be made but at last it was, and got scooped out of the machine into bowls. It was quite delicious and stupendously worth the pain and effort that had gone into it.

All Larry's friends looked at me askance. If you had never known what that word meant you would know if you saw the way they stared at me. Some of them were wondering what I was doing there, but most of them thought they knew. It took me a while to work it out but I was helped one day when a couple of them said quietly and laughingly to Larry as we were driving off in the car, 'You know she's jail-bait, Larry?'. This meant that I was underage and that he could be jailed for sleeping with me. He was not sleeping with me, but he didn't seem to mind if people believed he was, and did nothing to disabuse the people who thought so.

We visited many people. Larry seemed to have an endless supply of cousins on every rung of the social ladder. We met his mother, who had married at thirteen and given birth to him a year later, and from whom he was rather distanced for some reason, and two of his brothers, one of whom had an endless supply of moonshine liquor which he made himself in a still in the woods. One day we visited a decidedly impecunious family of relatives who lived in a shack on the side of the mountain. The mother was called Miss Mamie Pearl Duckworth Golightly, and her son, who seemed rather simple, entertained us by picking the banjo and singing mountain ditties. We went to visit them on hired ponies, rather an uncomfortable experience for me, as, though I could just about ride, I had never sat on a Western saddle before. On the way back we heard a tremendous shuffling in the trees and Larry said it was probably a bear.

All the family and friends in Black Mountain were friendly, but none overtly so. The thing was that Larry seemed like a bit of an oddity in the family. This had more to do with his literary leanings and his love for Europe than with his sexuality. Certainly he was gay, or rather bisexual, but then so, as it turned out, were practically all the people we met. Everyone seemed to sleep with everyone else, regardless of class, race, or gender. Larry said to me one day, half jokingly, 'The thing about niggers is that they can all be <u>had</u>'. On one occasion he arranged for me to go out with a girl cousin of his, a year or so older than me. She had a car and took me out sightseeing. She was shorthaired and chunky and I did not really warm to her. On the way home she said to me:

*Are you on the committee?*
*On the committee? What committee?*

Somehow she made me understand what the expression meant — it meant was I gay. She didn't use this word — I think what she said was, Do you swing both ways? I explain that I did not, and she expressed deep surprise. Everyone else she knew did, including, naturally, herself.

Certainly Larry seemed to have a very high proportion of gay friends. I did not mind this at all, or even find it particularly surprising, since I seemed to have been surrounded by homosexuals for most of my life. I didn't know any gay women, though, and I actually took very much to Larry's two closest women friends, a couple of lesbian librarians who lived in Ashville: they seemed warm, friendly, and nurturing, as well as funny and intelligent.

Ashville was the nearest big town and we often went in there to visit a (straight) married couple. The husband was a lawyer and also what I learned to call a redneck. In their house a great deal of alcohol was consumed, and I got to like something called a Tom Collins and also took to Bourbon, in a long glass with ice and lemon. The husband was shockingly racist and Larry enjoyed encouraging him though I hoped he did not share these ideas — he said that black people had to have separate restaurants and cinemas because they smelled so bad.

In this house Larry seemed more comfortable, and here he talked openly about his sexuality. It transpired that, though he also liked women, what he had to do from time to time was go out and pick up truck drivers for sex. In fact in the middle of my stay he disappeared for a couple of days for this very purpose. I found this rather distressing and confusing, although the Ashville friends seemed to accept it and take it for granted, and nobody was ever shocked or judgmental. I had not been brought up to be judgmental either: although my parents were rather good and moral, many of their friends lived highly irregular lives. However what confused me about this particular business was that, just before the truck-driver expedition, Larry had started to make love to me. Not, I hasten to say, to take me to bed, as even he was probably aware that this would be rather irresponsible under the circumstances. But on a drive out into the mountains one day he had started to kiss me, and after that he did it quite a lot, usually before I went to bed at night. The result was that I was deeply in love with him. So when he went off to find the truck-drivers I was devastated. The night he was due back I stood by the window in my room in the dark for hours, waiting for his car lights to appear so that I would know he was home.

When he came back, Larry came up with a plan. He thought we should get married. Not only that, but we would then go to Florida, where a lot of rich old men were to be found, and he would pass me off as an English aristocrat and sell me to a millionaire. We would then be able to live off the proceeds. This sounds completely ludicrous and I can't believe at this distance in time that he was really serious. But the plan was much discussed during the last part of my stay, and I was desperately trying to think what exactly I would say to my parents about it all. Luckily I never did have to tell them, as Larry appeared one day to say he had had a change of plan. He was going to go into a monastery. And so he did, though he came out again some time later and did, rather briefly and disastrously, marry someone else.

So I travelled back as planned. It was a solitary journey, up to New York on the Greyhound Bus, feeling rather bereft. When I climbed onto the bus at Ashville there was nowhere to sit apart from one seat next to a large and motherly looking black lady, so I made myself comfortable there. Before the bus left, the driver made his way down to me and started incomprehensibly apologising to me profusely. At last I understood that it was because I had to sit next to a black person. As we travelled through the night, I fell asleep and woke next morning to find I had spent all night with my head resting on her large and soft shoulder. She smiled at me a lot, but we never spoke.

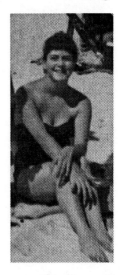

In New York I was actually met this time, by George Goetschius's aged parents, who took me back for a soothing few days in their suburban house. With his sister we went to the beach on Labor Day, and a photograph taken there shows me looking smooth and plump, young and innocent, though I was a little less innocent than I had been a couple of months earlier. The Goetschiuses saw me onto my return ship, the SS America. It was full of American students on their

*Labor Day on the beach*

way to Europe for Fulbright scholarships. It was a jolly voyage, completely different from the one coming over. There were parties every night, and I managed to continue drinking my favourite Tom Collins. I made friends with a clever, ugly, Jewish boy and we sat up late into the night talking. The sea was rough but I was unfazed by it. One night as we sat on deck there was a huge full moon, the biggest I had ever seen. As the ship tipped and dipped, the moon appeared to shoot up and down the sky, as if the ship was still and only the moon was moving.

# 10

I had to find something to do for a year before trying LAMDA again. Anything but the theatre was unthinkable – it never occurred to me then, or for many years afterwards, that there was anywhere else to work. Soon after I came back from America a perfect opportunity presented itself. John Dexter, who I knew because he was one of the assistant directors at the Court, was asked to direct two plays — a double bill — by Willis Hall, at the Lyric Hammersmith, and he needed an assistant stage manager. Would I like to do the job? I certainly would. On the first day of rehearsals I met the other ASM, a dark, skinny boy from Cardiff called Peter Gill. Working for John Dexter was a lot of fun. He had, even then, the reputation of being unbelievably unpleasant to his actors and others involved with his productions but to me, and to Peter, he was invariably sweet and gentle. I enjoyed the challenge of being an efficient ASM though really all I was was a runner: I had to get the props onto the stage at the right time, ring telephone bells and other dogsbody-ish activities. Having been frittering my

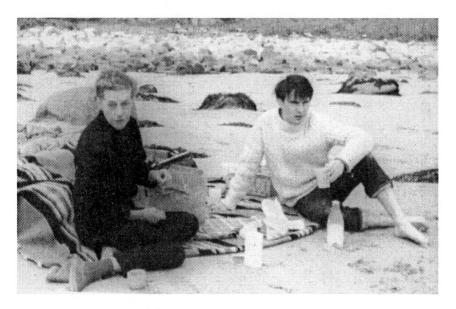

*Peter Gill with Sophie on a beach*

time away for so long, uncertain what I really should be doing with my life, I felt at last that I had come home to the place I really wanted to be. The cast, which included Jill Bennett and Paul Daneman, was universally kind and encouraging and the whole experience was, for me at least, a hugely successful one.

The best thing of all about it was getting to be friends with Peter Gill. A couple of years older than me, he had almost the same birthday — we were both Virgos — and we certainly seemed to have many things in common, including a sense of humour. He was, as he pointed out to me recently, my first real grown-up friend. We seemed to hit it off right away and before long we were inseparable, spending almost all our time together.

Peter used to come and spend his days at Lower Mall and quickly found his way to my mother's heart, as she did to his. We would sit for hours in the kitchen watching Sophie draw and smoke, drinking strong tea and making endless plates of scrambled eggs on toast, which appeared to be our staple diet. We would go to exhibitions, and plays, and films. There always seemed to be a party to go to, frequently enlivened by the appearance of a collection of people we knew as the drinking actors: Peter O'Toole, Stanley Baker and Michael Caine.

Above all, when we were not at Lower Mall, we would spend most of our time at John Dexter's flat in Castlenau, just on the other side of Hammersmith Bridge. We enjoyed John's company and liked his caustic sense of humour though he treated both of us with great gentleness. In his flat at any given time there would always be a large collection of boys. Not children (though, as we discovered later, John would have been happy if so), but boy actors, youthful looking chaps in their late teens and early twenties. He liked to be surrounded by them even if they were not gay but straight, as in fact most of them were. They were all rather attractive so it was pleasant to be in their company.

The conversation was always very interesting and informative and I learned a lot about homosexuality and the sort of things people did, or wished they could do. Relatively innocent and inexperienced, I liked hanging around with these kind of people as it was unthreatening for me. And I loved Peter Gill, but it was a love that was unrequited in the sense of anything physical taking place, though I've no doubt that Peter did love me deeply as a friend. One day in the hall at Lower Mall, just as he was leaving he kissed me goodbye and by chance or by design (mine) his kiss landed on my lips. He stepped back quickly and said quietly, 'A chaste kiss once in a while…'. He never spoke to me of his own sexual preferences but it was not difficult to guess that they did not include girls, although I heard a rumour that he had briefly gone out with Sandra Lousada.

I did sometimes wish that we could have more than a chaste kiss once in a while, but it was a happy time for me. We were good companions and it was great not to be lonely and feel a bit like an outcast, and it filled my life in a wholly positive way. The other thing that was good at this time was the way my friendship with Peter and John and Bill Gaskill fed into my mother's life. As time went on Lower Mall was filled more and more with people sitting in the kitchen drinking tea and eating scrambled eggs and playing cards. Bill and I and Peter and Bill's friend Donald Harris used to play for money, and Bill would slowly up the stakes until I was forced to drop out: I hated to lose and so was never much of a gambler. But Bill and whoever he had managed to rope in would go on and on playing, for frightening sums like half a crown or even ten shillings, until someone was completely broke. Bill also liked to make us play a game of identifying the first lines of Shakespeare's plays, something I had done with my mother since I was a child. Sophie was good at it but I was even better, for some unknown reason, even if I had never seen or read the plays in question.

It was at a party that I had gone to with John Dexter and Peter and some of the boy actors that I first met Chris Sandford. He was indeed a boy actor himself, having started at the Corona Stage School at a very young age. Now he was twenty-one and was appearing in an Agatha Christie play in the West End. He also turned out to have been in a brief relationship with Sandra Lousada. While not strictly beautiful he was extremely attractive and very charming, tall and skinny, with long fair hair that constantly flopped into his eyes. He was elegant and talented, a good actor but also able to play the guitar and sing and dance. Although he had also been brought up in a theatrical background, his was very different from mine: his father was a musical-hall comedian called Sandy Sandford whose name could be seen every week in a little box on the back of the Stage newspaper.

So there we all were at the party, and Chris and I seemed to like each other

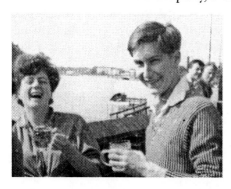

*With Chris on Lower Mall*

very much. He told me later that he had been attracted to me because of my pony-tail, and had been a little put out when it proved to be a false one, which I wore because my hair was too wiry and curly to hang properly. In any case before the evening was over he had asked for my telephone number and a few days afterwards he telephoned and asked me to go out with him. I could hardly believe this was true.

Despite the many kisses I had never been out on a real date, and had no sense of myself as remotely attractive. But I went with dignity. He took me to a party, and on the way back home on the tube we kissed. When we got back to Lower Mall I said he could sleep in the spare room — George's old room — and we kissed some more and then we got into the bed and I lost my virginity without a thought except one of relief and pleasure that it was about time for this to happen.

So at last I had a real boyfriend, and after this first evening we were an established couple. Chris would come to the house in the afternoons when my mother was at work, or stay the night after the play, and we spent most of our time in bed together. Whether my mother knew this was happening or not I have no idea, though I think she must have guessed. Certainly, though, we never discussed it. I am not sure how much she or my father really approved of Chris. He was a good actor, which would have endeared him to George, but he was not, you might say, of our world and did not really all that much enjoy the company of people like Peter and Bill, preferring to have me to himself, I think. He seemed to think me very beautiful, which was good for morale though I never entirely believed it when he called me a 'rare beauty'.

Peter did not, I believe, feel very pleased about my relationship with Chris. He and I still spent a lot of time together when Chris was not around. I continued to love Peter although I was at the same time besotted with Chris and what we used to get up to together. For a long time Peter did not know that Chris and I were sleeping together, and perhaps he was a bit shocked when I finally let on that we were. In a way, perhaps, he was jealous, not of the sex, but of the fact that instead of wanting to spend all my time with him I now had another interest in my life. It was a change, and change is always difficult.

During all this, throughout the break-up with my father and the trauma associated with it, my mother never stopped working. There was a short period of panic just after he left when she thought her life had come to an end on all fronts, work included, and during this time she managed to keep going by designing dresses for Berketex. She also did some textile designs for Courtaulds. In fact, however, the theatre and film work soon took over again. During the year when I went to America and met Chris, for instance, she designed Pinero's *The Magistrate* at the Old Vic in March, *The Aspern Papers* at the Queen's and an opera, *Tannhaüser*, at Sadlers Wells in December. She also designed a production of *Rosmersholm* , directed by my father, at the Court. An undated letter from George seems to refer to this – it's a little formal, but has a genuine warmth which is pleasing :

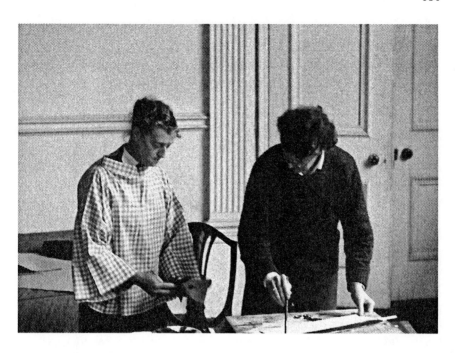

*Sophie and Percy working*

*Dearest Soph*
*Thank you so much for all your care and skill and hard work....It's nice too having*
*you back here, altho' it's for 2 1/2d!*
*Love, G*

Four productions seems quite good going, but the following year she did
the costumes for no less than seven stage plays, including Rattigan's *Ross*
(Haymarket) and Bolt's *Man for all Seasons* (Globe) and also for a film, the
celebrated Woodfall production *Saturday Night and Sunday Morning*, directed
by Karel Reisz.

Her fears that she would be ostracised by directors more closely associated
with my father proved groundless, especially in the case of Tony Richardson
and his Woodfall associates. *Saturday Night* was followed the next year by *A
Taste of Honey*, which Tony directed himself. This was filmed mainly at the old
Royal Court scenic workshops in Park Walk, at the end of the Kings Road,
a location that held many memories for Sophie since it was the very same
place where she, Percy and Liz had gone to art college so many years earlier.
The year after she worked for Tony again on Alan Sillitoe's *The Loneliness
of the Long Distance Runner*, and her final Woodfall film, directed by Lindsay
Anderson, was *This Sporting Life*. What these directors had recognised, I

think, was her particular talent for authenticity: even in films such as these, with contemporary working-class settings, she was able to dress the actors so that they appeared both wholly real and entirely in character.

As for my relationship with my mother, it had improved a bit since my angry and resentful earlier teenage years, but I was, I know, less sympathetic to her than I might have been. Percy told me quite recently that I had upset Sophie desperately by saying to her one day that I was not surprised my father had left her: 'You were too nice to him'. If I did say so, I have successfully blotted out that particular memory, but I certainly do remember thinking and feeling something of the kind. She seemed so soft, so dependent, so acquiescent, and I wanted her to fight back, to tell him to go to hell, to get on with her own life and forget him. But I fear she had loved him for too many years to be able to do that. He was her life and I suppose had always been since that first meeting in Oxford all those years ago, and she simply was not able to cut that out of herself. It is very sad to read the letters that he wrote to her in the years after they had parted. They are invariably kind and considerate, but there is usually a rather distant formality about them that must have been hard to take. 'Dear Sophie', or 'My dear Sophie', they begin, and they end dutifully enough with 'love to you both', but there is little warmth in them. There are indications that she was expressing her pain in letters to him ('I will answer your letter later. It is full of misapprehensions'), but her letters, perhaps thankfully, have not survived. I myself appear in his letters from time to time, as a rather minor character – 'I will look after Harriet. She must join me at the theatre for the show' – 'I am going to take Harriet to the Vic with me on Tues night – Royal visit – It'll probably be ghastly but she might enjoy it!'. Reading these, I wonder how he felt about me at this time. Guilty, no doubt, and perhaps rather shy. Perhaps he thought that I was angry with him for leaving Sophie. I am now trying to think whether in fact I was, but I think not. Hurt, cast off and unloved, yes, but angry no.

All in all I do not congratulate myself on the way I treated my mother for the last years of her life. However I am pleased that I was indirectly responsible for the fact that she was, at least, surrounded by people who increasingly came to love her and depend on her. Tony had moved out by this time, married Vanessa Redgrave, and installed himself in a house in St Peter's Square just down the road. Our top-floor flat was still inhabited by George Goetschius, who now lived with Donald Howarth. On the day of Tony's final departure, the two of them had barricaded Donald in the studio with those of

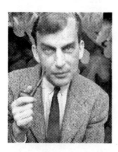

*George Goetschius*

George's belongings they had been afraid Tony might make off with: he sat in there trembling, listening to Tony and his friends rattling the door handle, unable to get into the room. George loved my mother deeply as did Peter Gill, who had ceased to be a frequent overnight guest and become an established lodger.

One thing that is good to remember among all this sadness is that Sophie never lost her sense of humour. She and I were devoted fans of Peter Cook and Dudley Moore, and laughed ourselves into agony at a sketch, the content of which I have mostly forgotten, in which Cook, describing his mother I think, said, 'She could break a swan's neck with a blow of her arm'. Peter Gill was hugely entertaining and the three of us were often hysterical with laughter as we played some extremely silly games, such as Peter's creation of various stock Welsh types in hats: our all-time favourite was the pugnacious collier, his hat pulled right down and his lower lip curled over, who could have us in giggles in an instant.

After the run of the Willis Hall plays was finished I was on the loose again for a while, but I luckily managed to get myself another job soon afterwards. A play by the surrealistically comic writer N.F. Simpson (known as Wally), *One Way Pendulum*, had been so successful at the Court that it was decided to transfer it to the West End, and a booking was made at the Criterion Theatre in Piccadilly Circus. Again an ASM was needed and again I managed to get the job. Again I was the second ASM, the chief one being Donald Harris, a dark and handsome New Zealander who was involved in a relationship with the director, Bill Gaskill. Our stage manager was a Junoesque beauty only a few years older than me called Jocelyn Tawse. I enormously enjoyed working on the play because I found it so extremely funny: we all did. Wally Simpson's humour was so bizarre. The play concerned the Groomkirbys, a happily dysfunctional family — their daughter, Sylvia, complaining ceaselessly because her arms were not long enough and she had to bend down to make them reach her knees, and envying apes for their better endowment in this department ('Apes are bending all the time, Sylvia, as well you know'), their son up in the bedroom teaching speak-your-weight machines to sing the Hallelujah Chorus. One of my jobs was to make the food that was eaten on stage every night by the actress playing the old lady who came in every day to eat up the leftovers: jelly and instant mashed potato, which she was called upon to shovel down in large quantities. The climax of the play was a trial scene — the entire courtroom being set up in the family living room.

*Judge: Does he have any coloured blood?*
*Mrs Groomkirby: Well, he does have one or two bottles upstairs in the bathroom.*

The ending was triumphant, as the speak-your-weight machines finally learned to sing Handel, and my final job was to turn on the tape that belted it out at full volume.

The run at the Criterion started in the spring. I had been going out with Chris for perhaps six months and we had hit a rather sticky patch for some reason. I remember Chris's father, who was a very warm and kindly man, advising us that perhaps we had been seeing a bit too much of each other, as we were relatively still so young. We didn't want to break up, but we decided to ease off a bit. During the run of the play I had a brief but rather passionate flirtation with Donald Harris, though it never progressed beyond kissing in a large armchair in a dressing room, and once in a taxi travelling towards Hammersmith. Oddly enough I also had one with Bill Gaskill, but perhaps this was a little earlier — we had started kissing like mad at a party and also once did so on the underground, which he told me pleased him a lot because, not given to having affairs with women, this was something he had not had the opportunity to do before.

During the run of the play I got to be rather good friends with Jocelyn Tawse, the stage manager, and as the run was coming to an end she and I decided to go on holiday together. I had been earning the grand sum of £12 a week and, since I was living at home, I had managed to save enough to pay for such a thing. I was very excited, as this would be my first proper holiday independent of my parents – Rome and North Carolina had not seemed quite to fit that definition . My mother had some friends, people she had stayed with a year or two earlier, whose names were Sam and Daphne Ainley and who ran a sort of high-class theatrical pension in Majorca. So she arranged for Jocelyn and me to go there for our holiday.

The Ainleys were quite a couple. Sam was the son of a famous, long-dead actor by the name of Henry Ainley, a man with a reputation. He supposedly had a string of mistresses and dozens of illegitimate offspring. My mother used to tell a story of an aristocratic lady at a dinner party being asked, 'Do you know Henry Ainley?', to which she had replied, in a Lady Bracknell-ish sort of voice, 'Know him? He is the father of two of my children!'.

As my mother did, to do her justice, warn us before we left, Sam had to a great extent taken on the mantle of his father. He was thought to be relatively safe, however, because he was married to Daphne Rye, who was large and rather scary. So off Jocelyn and I went to Palma, on the plane, and soon found ourselves at the Ainleys' lovely villa, perched on the edge of the coast about half an hour away from the town. We were not the only guests: also staying there were an actor, Daniel Massey, and his girlfriend, the very striking actress Adrienne Corri, who had a beautiful body and masses of red hair. They seemed to us astonishingly sophisticated and made us feel like a couple of kids, which indeed in a sense we were. I was seventeen, and Jocelyn in her early twenties. Everyone was, on the surface at least, very kind and welcoming, but we had the feeling that Dan and Adrienne secretly rather despised us.

A day or so after we arrived we were taken to what was supposed to be one of the high points of the holiday, a bullfight in Palma. This was meant to be a great treat but I hated it, finding it horrifying and upsetting. Apart from this outing we spent our time at the house in our swimming costumes, sunning ourselves on the terrace or lying on the tiny private beach, and eating large amounts of Daphne's elaborate meals. A few days later a second bullfight was announced, but I really did not want to go. Sam said he was not keen either and would stay home and keep me company.

Once everyone had driven off in the car, Sam lost no time in taking me into the living room and starting to kiss me. I had been rather expecting this from things he had said, but I felt distinctly ambivalent about it as I had Chris waiting for me at home. Luckily I did not have to make any major decisions as he soon stopped again and said he was sorry, but although when I arrived he had been very anxious to get me into bed, he was now unable to do so: 'I have fallen deeply in love with your friend'. Rather relieved, I said this was quite all right, and we spent a companionable day together.

Within the next couple of days Sam managed to contrive a situation where he was on his own with Jocelyn and the two of them did indeed end up in bed together. There was remarkably little secrecy about it, and we assumed that this must be something that he and Daphne accepted as part of their relationship. We could not have been more wrong. As soon as the facts became known, Dan and Adrienne and Daphne refused to speak to us at all, and when we were in our bedroom we would hear the three of them outside on the terrace discussing our lack of morals in loud and harsh voices. Sent to Coventry, we skulked around for the last few days of our holiday, keeping out of everyone's way as much as possible.

Just before we were due to leave, Sam asked Jocelyn to stay on for a few days, and she agreed to do so. So the two of them took me to the airport and I made my lonely way back to London while they disappeared off to some secret love-nest. I saw her when she came back, glowing, and she told me that he had been a wonderful lover, but we were too shy to discuss exactly what it was that they had done together. I did remember him saying publicly on the terrace at the villa, 'I've only got a little winkle, but I know how to use it'. As far as I know she never saw him again, but the two of us lost touch after that episode. I was rather glad to get back to normal life again. It had been a strange adventure, and an interesting demonstration of how innocent and yet how open to suggestions we both were.

Soon after I got back from Majorca it was time once again to audition for LAMDA, and this time I was accepted. Unfortunately I could not let go of a deeply rooted suspicion that this was because I was George Devine's daughter. In any case, full of excitement and trepidation, I started there in September, having just turned eighteen. Now I had a strange experience. Acting was what I had been longing to do with all my heart and soul, ever since I was a tiny child pretending to be Titania on the Old Vic Stage. Catherine and I had frequently put on plays for our parents. Every summer we had spent at Stratford I had imagined myself as Juliet, as Cordelia, as Desdemona, learning the parts and acting them out in the secrecy of my bedroom. At school I always seemed to be given leading parts, and had felt I had acquitted myself pretty well in them. For some reason or other, though, once I got to LAMDA I froze up, and I never really managed to unfreeze.

This was not because I did not enjoy the classes — I enjoyed them a lot. We had a wonderful voice teacher called Iris Warren, who had taught at the London Theatre Studio before the war. She taught us to do what she called 'centring' our voices. This was an amazing trick. All you had to do was stand up, place your hand on your diaphragm, and say 'Huh-hurm-ah'. But you had to find out how to say this, not as you would normally do from your throat or even your chest, but from a place deep inside that Iris and her assistant Kristin Linklater told us was called your centre. None of us could do it at first but slowly, over the days and weeks, one by one we caught on to how to do it. When we finally did, it was great. It turned out to be true what Iris and Kristin said, that once you found your centre you would never lose it. No more problems with projection, no strain, no effort at all, and you could use this centred voice in all your work, speaking or singing.

Iris and Kristin had, they said, developed this technique partly because they were practising a kind of meditation that was taught by someone called Maharishi Mahesh Yogi. It was called Transcendental Meditation. One day when I was at LAMDA they told us that he was coming to London and would be giving a talk at the Albert Hall. They invited us to go along and a number of my friends did go. I, however, refused. I did not see the point and thought the whole thing sounded stupid, spooky and altogether too foreign for my liking. This was an interesting reaction, considering the fact that eight or so years later I would learn to do this meditation and continue to do it for the rest of my life.

Each year's intake at LAMDA was quite small, and we all became very close and friendly. I had various flirtations, but still considered myself attached to Chris, though things had been distinctly wobbly for a while. Earlier that year we had gone on the Aldermaston march, by now an annual event, and I had lost him in Trafalgar Square at the end. I sought him out in Soho, where he liked to frequent folk clubs, and to my horror spotted him disappearing into one of them hand in hand with a rather beautiful redhead. It really was like being stabbed in the heart. However, after a rather distant and painful summer, he was called up for his National Service and asked me, on his first leave, if I would get engaged. Of course I said yes.

A good friend of mine on the acting course at LAMDA was a splendid Canadian girl, Carolyn Jones. She was tall and dark and seemed to me to be a very strong person whose company I always enjoyed. She had a flat in Earls Court, not far from LAMDA, and we spent many happy afternoons there. She had an American boyfriend and was much preoccupied with the subject of birth control. Having solved the problem for herself, she packed me off to the lady doctor she had found, who asked me a lot of what I found rather embarrassing questions. However I ended up by coming away with a rather messy and awkward device called a Dutch Cap, which would make things with Chris easier and pleasanter in the long run. He would come back from his army camp on occasional weekends and sit in the back room at Lower Mall polishing his boots with black polish, a candle and lots of spit. I used to darn his army socks, feeling a bit ambivalent about such enforced domesticity.

I had by this time lost some weight but I still was far from the slender creature I would have liked to be. Carolyn and I were constantly dieting but we were hideously weak-willed. One day we bought ourselves a bag of sweets with the foolish intention of having one each a day. We kept dipping in and then feeling horribly guilty. At last Carolyn said, 'For goodness sake let's finish these off, then they won't be around to tempt us any more'.

My best friend at LAMDA, though, was not on the acting course at all. Her name was Georgina Shaw, and she was training to be a stage manager. Even chubbier than I was, highly intelligent, extremely witty, Georgina was very emotionally confused. This was largely a result of how her parents treated her. Her father was a diplomat but he did not extend his diplomacy to his daughter. One day he came to pick her up from our house after the weekend and said to my mother, 'Has my great lump of a daughter been a nuisance to you?', which made Sophie absolutely furious. Georgina and her sister and brother had been brought up in all sorts of exotic places like Libya and Kenya and her mother, whose nickname was Nutkin, had taken rather heavily to gin, presumably a result of the pressures of life as a diplomat's wife. She would often be found in the kitchen of their sizeable country house, sipping away at a large tumbler of what looked like water, but wasn't, as she cooked. She also wrote rather successful detective stories.

Somehow or other Georgina had got to know a flat full of extremely interesting men who lived not far from LAMDA in Philbeach Gardens. Most of them were homosexual, which was fine by me as most people I knew were anyway. The flat belonged to Jeremy Kingston, a writer who lived with an actor from Pakistan called Rashid Karapiet. They seemed to have a large circle of interesting friends including a wild-eyed poet, Harry Fainlight, and also Christopher Isherwood. Best fun of all was Michael Fish, a young man — hardly more than a boy — who worked at a grand men's shirt shop in Jermyn Street called Turnbull and Asser, although one day in the not too far distant future he would have his own shop and sell shirts to people like the Rolling Stones.

These people were just visitors to the flat but Jeremy and Rashid also had a lodger, who alone among the whole lot of them was not in fact gay. An architect turned furniture designer, his name was Peter Key and he was twenty-eight years old, which was ten years older than I was. I thought him very good-looking, blond and blue-eyed, with a body that I later came to think of as being like that of Michaelangelo's David. Quite how he had ended up living in a household such as this was a bit of a mystery, but he was very easy with everyone and they were all very open with him even though he did not join in their sexual activities.

Philbeach Gardens rapidly became the centre of my social life: days at LAMDA, evenings at Philbeach Gardens. We seemed to spend most of our time there playing games. These were sometimes card games like Knock, a satisfyingly noisy game that required you to bang on the table when you were down to your last card. Another game we never got tired of was a form of charades in which you have a phrase or title to mime to

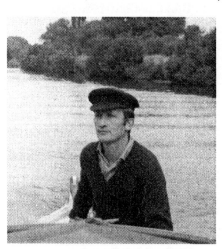

*Peter Key in Percy's boat*

your team, who have to guess as many as possible. We played this for hours with great hilarity, though I was rather put out one day when I was trying to act out something or other and Georgina's loud whisper came flying across the room: 'She's usually very good at this!'.

I enjoyed being at Philbeach Gardens and most of all I enjoyed the fact that Peter Key seemed to have taken a fancy to me. With Chris away at Richmond in Yorkshire, and so involved with the spitting and polishing of his boots when I did see him, I found it difficult to feel as committed as I should. And Peter Key was very charming and persuasive, so much so that kisses at a party were not, as they usually seemed to be, the end of it all. Before too much time had passed I found myself staying the night in Peter's bed at Philbeach Gardens.

# 11

Sleeping with Peter Key turned out to be very enjoyable, and it had the added charm of being secret and forbidden. Well, it was hardly secret since Georgina and Jeremy and Rashid and all the Philbeach Gardens people knew all about it, but it was secret from Chris and from my family. And so I went on for many months, leading this rather shabby double life, until at last my mother confronted me with a straight question and I saw no point in not confessing.

Sophie was upset and disappointed in me. This was not so much because she thought I should marry Chris, as she was fond of him but I do not believe she thought he was right for me. Her disappointment was because of the way I had been carrying on for so long behind his back. 'You must tell Chris at once', she said, and I saw that indeed I must. Sophie was essentially such a good and honest woman and I had just broken the fundamental rule of her morality: that nothing is wrong unless it hurts someone else. So the next weekend when he turned up on leave I made myself tell him. It was hard to do, but I felt better for having done it. After his initial rather tearful reaction, though, he and Peter went off to the pub together and got drunk, leaving me and Sophie rather surprisedly alone at home. Luckily soon after he got back to Richmond he started going out with the beautiful daughter of his commanding officer and when his National Service was finished the two of them got married.

So then Peter Key and I were officially a couple. Apart from that, life went on pretty much as usual. LAMDA featured very largely in my life, obviously, but I was beginning to fear that after all I might not be going to be such a great actress. I continued to enjoy the classes — fencing, falling off chairs, dashing across the room and diving into forward rolls on rubber mats, dancing like Fred Astaire and Ginger Rogers — but when it came to the acting itself I just seemed not to do it all that well. I had plenty of chances to shine. I played Natasha, the awful wife of Andrey in *The Three Sisters*, all in pink with frizzy hair. I was Hermia in the *Midsummer Night's Dream*, a part I had longed to play for years, but I didn't gel at all with the rather stodgy Indian who was my Lysander. I hugely enjoyed a Jacobean shocker, *'Tis Pity She's a Whore*, playing opposite a boy called John Samson (who I had managed to charm on my first day at LAMDA simply by looking up at him in a certain way) as an incestuous brother and sister. Whatever I did, however, somehow other people always seemed to be the stars and I felt like the inferior article. I never seemed to manage to lose my self-consciousness.

Thinking about it now after all these years I seriously wonder how much this had to do with the fact that, throughout my two years at LAMDA, my father never once came to see me perform. George Goetschius has told me recently how shocked he and other people in the Lower Mall circle were at his staying away. I have no doubt that it was because he was afraid I was not going to be very good, and though I did not think of it in those terms at the time, it was a self-fulfilling prophecy. It was at around this time that I started to feel more and more rejected by him, and his apparent lack of interest in my acting career was a huge factor, I am sure. Other children of theatre people could be assured that their parents would employ them or at least see to it that they got employed, but the story in our family was that my father was completely opposed to nepotism and so would go out of his way not to give me work. The trouble with this view was that other people tended to think, rightly or wrongly, that I could not be much good if even my own father would not give me a job.

Finally my time at LAMDA came to an end and it was time for what amounted to my graduation performance. This was certainly, as far as I was concerned, the best thing I had ever done. It was a one-acter, and a one-person piece, an American play the title and author of which have both escaped me. All I can remember was the opening music ('Why should I have spring fever/When it isn't even spring?') and me, playing a rather foolish and neurotic young woman, found reclining on a bed as the curtain rose. I think the reason it went well was because of the director, who was Prunella Scales, another ex-Old Vic School person and a wonderful comedy actress. The best thing about working with her was that she took me absolutely seriously and directed me as if I did have some talent, which immediately brought out whatever modicum of it I did possess. But that was the end, and after it I was cast out into the world and had to try to find myself a job. Given my father's resolution, there would be nothing for me at the Court.

Although this is hardly an excuse for apparently casting me off, George was having a particularly difficult time of it. It was now six years since the euphoric launch of the English Stage Company, and the history of those six years had been a history of battles, disappointments and compromises. Certainly new writers of real stature had emerged: Arnold Wesker, Ann Jellicoe, Edward Bond, John Arden. But the theatre never made money and frequently lost it — John Arden's *The Happy Haven* lost £14,757, for example, and his *Sergeant Musgrave's Dance* , which has now become an A-level text, lost £5,820. These were huge sums of money in those days. To keep things afloat and to keep the ESC Council happy, the company occasionally put on supposed crowd-pleasers in the way of classic revivals. Sometimes these worked well. *The Country Wife* was a huge success and transferred to New York, and *The Entertainer, Rosmersholm* and *One Way Pendulum* did well in the West End, for example. But each new play that was put on had to run the gamut of the ESC Council and those struggles, together with the fact that, despite having a talented collection of Assistant Artistic Directors, George seemed to have to do most of the work himself, had exhausted my father almost beyond endurance.

His stress and fatigue had come to a head while I was in my first year at LAMDA. His friend Nigel Dennis was commissioned to write a third play, *August for the People*, in which Rex Harrison (who had already appeared at the Court the previous year in Chekhov's *Platonov*) agreed to play the leading part. This seemed like a recipe for success, but in the event the play was perceived as being both right-wing and badly written, at least in the final act. Dennis and Harrison fell out, and Lindsay Anderson headed an anti-Dennis demonstration on the steps of the Court on the first night. Rex Harrison bought himself out of the production after two weeks and the play was forced to close. Nigel Dennis blamed my father for the debacle, and George, the strain of all this added to the accumulation of stress built up over the past several years hard work, succumbed to a nervous breakdown. I imagine that the stress of separating from my mother, notwithstanding his great happiness at being with Jocelyn, was also a contributing factor.

So all this was going on while I was struggling through my two years at LAMDA, and I suppose that makes it marginally easier to understand why he might not have had either the time or energy to come and see me acting in end of term productions. Harder to take and to explain away was his failure to include me in the riotous holiday that was the making of the

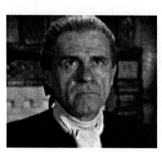

film *Tom Jones*, which happened in the summer after I finished at LAMDA. So much fun was had on that film by all concerned. Jocelyn designed the costumes, Tony Richardson directed, John Osborne wrote the screenplay, Sandra Lousada took the stills, and even Jenny Lousada, who was an artist rather than an actor, had a part in the film. But I was not invited. I minded that a lot. In fact it caused me excruciating pain. It only went to confirm what by now was an established

*George in* Tom Jones

feeling, that in moving on from Sophie my father had also moved on from me. I am sure if you had asked him about it he would not have seen it this way. Perhaps it never occurred to him that I would mind, and in any case he was not in charge of casting or directing. But it was, I suppose, a measure of our distance at this time. Somehow everything that happened between us now intensified my sense that I no longer mattered to him, and was not any more a part of his life. I have a vivid memory of one occasion when he appeared on the satirical TV show *That Was the Week That Was*, and gave tickets to me and Peter to be in the audience. I felt happy and proud to be there, and wanted to share those feelings with him afterwards. But instead he simply slipped away at the end without seeing us, perhaps to dine and drink with the rest of the cast, perhaps simply to go home to Jocelyn. I felt absolutely devastated, far more so than the occasion merited: all my feelings of rejection seemed suddenly to come to a head over what was surely just an oversight on his part.

Still, I had my own life and my own excitements. Peter Key and I had had our ups and downs, and had spilt up briefly in the spring of that year, but just before the end of my final term at LAMDA we had got back together and he had asked me to marry him. I was thrilled. Several of my friends seemed to be getting married, Lucinda Curtis — who had become a much-admired role model — included, and I loved the idea of having my own home. Having lost George, perhaps I was looking for a father-substitute, and Peter was ten years older, though he never behaved in a remotely fatherly way. In any case, the whole idea of marriage was exciting. We were to buy a houseboat on the Thames at Chelsea Reach which Peter, who possessed great carpentry skills, would convert for us to live in. It all sounded perfect to me. I was nineteen.

I can't say my parents seemed exactly thrilled, but they had never made any attempt to stop me doing anything I wanted to do and they were not about to start now. In fact I believe they were relieved that I would be taken care of by someone other than themselves. I don't mean that I think my mother wanted to get rid of me. Far from it. She was completely devoted to me although looking back I feel I did little to deserve her devotion, as I was at that time a selfish and ungrateful person, or so it sometimes seems to me now. But I think she felt that as she was tired and increasingly unwell it would be good if I had someone else to look out for me. And perhaps an older man seemed like a good bet.

That summer we rented a studio in St Ives and had a hilarious group holiday. As well as my mother and me, Georgina and Peter Gill came along, and Peter Key, though he managed only a part of it as he had to work. I think it was on this holiday that I started to wonder if I was really enough in love with Peter to make a marriage work. Not that there was anything wrong with him: he was sweet, funny, kind-hearted, generous, all the things you would hope for in a husband. It was just that some little voice inside was causing me momentary waverings, which I suppressed like mad by focusing on our plans for the boat and for the wedding itself.

So the plans went ahead. We decided to get married on Peter's birthday, 13 December, at Hammersmith Town Hall, and to have a party afterwards at Percy's studio in Earl's Court.

Invitations were printed out and sent off. We had a wedding list at Harvey Nichols, all Danish pottery and stainless steel cutlery and fashionable stacking glasses. I went to Mary Quant in the King's Road and bought an outfit: a black figured-velvet skirt and waistcoat, and a white crepe shirt with a very smart polo neck. But as the presents started to arrive my doubts got more and more pressing. One day, as Sophie and I were in the act of unpacking a white pottery teapot, I finally spoke.

*I don't think I ought to marry Peter Key. I don't think I'm in love with him.*
*Oh my darling,* (said Sophie), *everyone gets cold feet. Besides, we've sent out the invitations.*

This was, without doubt, the most uncharacteristic thing I ever heard her say. After all these years I am still puzzled by it. The only thing I can conclude is that she was anxious about my security. That is to say, she wanted to feel that I was going to be safe and well looked after.

One reason why she might have felt this was what had recently happened to her: in September of that year she had been admitted to hospital suffering from cancer of the uterus and had had a large, but apparently successful, operation. So all the way through the run-up to my wedding she was not only convalescing but also designing a production of a musical version of *Vanity Fair*. In fact as soon as the anaesthetic had worn off she was sitting up in bed drawing the designs for this rather unremarkable but large and demanding production. Anyone who thinks of Sophie as having been remotely weak should be given pause by this fact. Even though she presumably had an assistant, she recovered and began work again with almost frightening speed, somehow pressing on through the horrible chemotherapy which caused her hair to fall out, so that she had to wear a wig. It was during this period that she and Peter Gill went to see a play together. Meeting the author afterwards, Sophie told him quite untruthfully how much she had enjoyed it. Then, as they left the theatre, she turned to Peter and said, 'Everything about me is false: my teeth are false, my hair is false, and my opinions are false!'.

In any event, lacking my mother's support for my doubts about Peter Key, the wedding plans went ahead. Outwardly, the occasion itself went as well as such things usually do, I suppose. Hammersmith Town Hall is hardly the most romantic location you could imagine for such an event, and the ceremony, if you can call it that, seemed to me terribly dry and grey. Then we all decamped to Earl's Court Square and had a rather drunken party. My father came, looking rather uncomfortable as he always did in the presence of my mother. Glen came, and various members of the older generation. Then they all left and we kept on drinking, surrounded by people most of whom seemed to me to be Peter's friends rather than mine.

One new friend of mine was the actor David Warner, whom we had met in the Salisbury — the so-called actors' pub in St Martin's Lane — a couple of weeks earlier. He had been in *Tom Jones*, but had been unpopular with the rest of the cast, who seem to have identified him with Blifil, the unattractive and wicked character he was playing. When we first met him he was acting in a television play in which was also the young singer Bob Dylan. We had taken to each other rather a lot, and he and I and Peter had spent several evenings drinking together. At the wedding he sat in a corner, and then, when I went to see if he was alright, he burst into tears and said, 'If only we had met sooner — you could have been marrying me instead'. We could have met sooner, of course, if I had been invited to take part in *Tom Jones* , and perhaps if we had, I would indeed have married him instead. We had not, however, and I had married Peter Key.

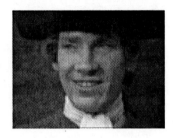

*David Warner in* Tom Jones

Marriage had not put an end to my attempts for an acting career. I was determined to make a success of it, despite, or because of, George's lack of interest and support. A number of people in my year at drama school had walked straight into jobs of various kinds, in rep, in TV, in films. I had not, but I had got myself an agent. Her name was Ros Chatto and she had signed me up in the last few weeks of the term. Her offices, overlooking Regent Street, were very plush, and once or twice a week I would go and sit there, chat a bit, and get sent occasionally for interviews, most of which came to nothing. Part of the trouble was, I am sure, the fact that I was still rather overweight, but I lacked the determination to do anything about this. I wonder, looking back, why Ros did not suggest that things might go better if I went on a diet, but she did not, and I simply carried on eating, feeling miserable about it but hoping it might perhaps go away, which it didn't. I compared myself unfavourably with one of Ros's other clients, Sarah Miles, who I met constantly at the office, often entwined with her boyfriend James Fox. He was a cousin of Georgina, who referred to him, as did his family and close friends, as Willie. She had taken me once to have a look at him when he had a temporary job at Fortnum and Mason. We had lurked about, gazing at him looking very handsome in his pinstripe trousers and tail coat. Now he was a star, and so was Sarah. The two of them seemed impossibly glamorous, and I heard stories of Sarah opening the door to visitors completely naked in order to show off her beautiful slender body.

In the end I did finally get a job, and it was in a film that Sarah and Willie were both going to play leading parts in. This was *The Servant*, written by Harold Pinter and starring Dirk Bogarde. The director was Joseph Losey, and instead of an audition I was invited to come and have breakfast with him in his little house in Chelsea. I thought him unbelievably attractive in a craggy, aged sort of way, and was amazed and delighted when I heard I had got the part.

Not that it was much of a part. There was a tiny scene of a minute or so in the film when Dirk Bogarde leaves the house in which he and Sarah Miles are manipulating their employer, to make a call from a telephone box. As he is phoning, a group of foolish girls come and tap on the glass and shout rudely at him to hurry up. One of those girls, plump and unattractively bleached blonde, is myself. I enjoyed doing it — well, I was working at last — but have never much enjoyed seeing myself in it.

Odd bits and pieces notwithstanding, I did not feel I was making much headway with my career. Then, not long after my wedding, Ann Jellicoe asked me if I would like a part in a Sunday night production she was directing at the Court. These Sunday shows, as they were called, were a great innovation at the theatre. Played without scenery and in the actors' own clothes, no-one taking salaries, they cost only about £100 to put on but gave writers and directors a chance to experiment with plays that were for some reason a little doubtful as main bill material. The one Ann wanted me to be in was written by Barry Reckord, the author of *Flesh to a Tiger*. Unlike his earlier Caribbean play it was set in London, and concerned the lives of four disaffected teenagers who were skiving off school. It was in fact called *Skyvers*.

Ann had cast an up and coming young actor, David Hemmings, to play the lead, and Annette Robertson, a tiny, talented girl who had been in *Tom Jones* and who got married to John Hurt on the day I married Peter, to play his girlfriend. The other couple were an actor called Philip Martin and me. The great thing about the rehearsal period was the fact that Ann, knowing George's views on employing me, had decided not to tell my father that I was going to be in the play. As we rehearsed in a hall some way from the theatre, and as he was as always ridiculously fraught with work, this was less of a problem than it sounds. So he actually came to the performance with no idea that I was to appear in one of the leading parts. If the play had not gone well, this would have been rather a mixed blessing.

Fortunately, though, it was a great success. I can hardly begin to express the feeling of pleasure I had when George came backstage after the show and said, clearly as surprised as I was, 'Darling, you were really good'. It was wonderful and amazing beyond belief. I felt like a real actress at last, and I felt validated because my father actually seems to recognise that I was.

Soon came some even better news. The play had been so successful that it was decided to put it on for a run. The original cast was invited to continue. So here at last was my chance to establish myself professionally, to get seen, and hopefully to move on to better things. However, something else was happening in my life. I had been married for three months by now and, predictably enough, I found I was pregnant. I was pleased about this, as it was, after all, the next thing to do. Lucinda, in whose footsteps I seemed to be following, had got married two weeks before me and now was going to have her first baby two weeks before me. But oh, what about *Skyvers*?

I had a long talk with Ann and we worked out dates. Although initially the pregnancy did not show, there was a delay before the play could be put on and by the time it started I would be four months pregnant, five and half by the end of the run. Alas, given the part I was to play, this was simply not on. I was dreadfully disappointed. My part went to Chloe Ashcroft, a niece of Peggy's, who played it perfectly well. For me, though, that seemed to be the end, more or less, of a great acting career.

Although I could not play the part in *Skyvers*, I could and did go to the classes my father ran for actors, both at the Court and at the Jeanetta Cochrane Theatre in Southampton Row. I carried on going to these right up to the end of my pregnancy, struggling with movement exercises despite my uncomfortable size. There were two different kinds of classes. One kind were for comedy acting of the sort my father had a predilection for: slapstick. He had always loved films by people like Laurel and Hardy, and music-hall comedy, and his own productions were often noted for his sure command of comic timing. Now he undertook to show actors how to do this.

Slapstick is a predominantly physical form of comedy and the great secret is for the actions to look completely unplanned and effortless while in fact they are planned down to the last split second of timing. They have to be or they will not work, and will certainly not get laughs. So there was a great deal of fun to be had, but hard work too, getting people on stage with ladders which swung round unpredictably, just avoiding hitting other people on the head, and other such technical problems.

I enjoyed the comedy classes but more than anything I enjoyed the other kind, the mask classes. These made a huge impression on all the participants and at least one play, John Arden's *The Happy Haven*, arose directly from the experience of working with the masks. Bill Gaskill tells a story about the very first class, in which my father gave a long and academic lecture about the origin and purpose of the comic, or half, mask, which meant, perhaps, less than he had hoped to the listeners. Then, right at the end, he turned his back for moment on the audience of writers, actors and directors, put on a mask and turned round again. As Bill puts it, this was a shocking and wonderful moment and seemed to have little to do with the theoretical talk he had just given.

Two kinds of mask can be used in theatre work and in the classes we experimented with both. There is the tragic mask, which covers the whole face and which is, obviously, a deeply serious mask, not caricatured at all. We used three: young, middle-aged and old. Because your mouth is covered in this mask you cannot speak, but for some reason every movement that you make takes on a huge significance. So you could act out a scene on your own — let's say a young girl comes in, sits down, reads a letter from her lover. If the actor is properly 'in' the mask and properly controlled, a tiny movement of the head will immediately indicate to the audience, leaving no room for doubt, whether the letter contains good news or bad. Unlike in comic-mask work, you do not look at yourself in the mirror in tragic masks, but you do spend some time gazing at the mask in your hands before you put it on. Tragic masks are hard to use well, as we all discovered, but everyone had a few successes and the effect was always extremely powerful. As I discovered a few years later when I learned to make masks myself, tragic masks are also difficult to make — in fact I never succeeded in making one with the proper absence of character.

Comic masks, as I also found out, are a great deal easier to construct. When I began doing this I discovered quickly how to build up, with plasticine on a blank plaster of Paris face, the right kind of grotesque or caricatured features. These I often based on the masks of the Italian Commedia del Arte, one of the main origins of this kind of mask work. In my father's classes we had a basket full of ready-made masks, and the class began with each actor going to the basket and choosing a mask for the day's work. There were characters of all kinds: foolish young girls, malevolent old men, lecherous old women. But the full character of the mask would not appear until it was on the actor's face. So the technique was this: you chose a mask, put it on, and stood in front of a long mirror gazing at yourself. You had to forget completely that this was Harriet, or that you were supposed to act. You had simply to see who it was that was looking back at you out of the mirror and then just be that person. Physical movements, a walk, gestures, came first and only much later did the mask find a voice.

This was not always easy, especially at first as we all had to lose our preconceptions. But when it worked it was quite wonderfully liberating. As it happened, my favourite mask was one of the very first to assume a fully-fledged character and to begin to speak, or at least to make noises. The mask was a pink and chubby one, with a pig-like snout for a nose and round red cheeks which gave it a permanent and extremely foolish smile, at least when it was on my face – another actor might produce a completely different character with the same mask. The name my character was given by the others in the class was Daisy Bum. This arose from her habit of shuffling across the room wiggling her behind in a rather childishly provocative way. At first it was just the movements, which, though it is hard to explain exactly why or how, simply arose from the experience of seeing her in the mirror. Then later she learned to make sounds, which never, in my case, developed into fully fledged Speech. Daisy just liked to make 'ooh' sounds, very high and piping ones, and could in fact make herself understood in a variety of modes by variations on this way of communicating.

There are all kinds of psychological theories about why half-masks work in the way they do. Basically, however, as was clear in my own case, they remove your sense of being yourself (overweight, unattractive) and allow you to enter into the consciousness of some other being. It is not surprising that this is liberating. Years later I was interested to read that the father of the Brontë sisters made his little daughters wear a mask when he was interrogating them about their successes and failures, and found it released answers which they would never have given unmasked.

So I was seeing my father quite regularly in the classes, though I was not treated as his daughter here but simply as a working member of the group. It is pleasant to record, though, that my pregnancy had brought us closer. It was a source of great pride and excitement for him. Not having seen me as a baby, he was hugely looking forward to being a grandfather. As well as at the mask classes, the other place I was seeing him quite often was on weekends at his newly acquired country cottage, Andrew's Farm, in Hampshire. Some of the money he and Jocelyn had earned from the film of *Tom Jones* had gone to buy and restore this lovely place, tucked away behind a wood in the middle of green fields. Buying it was, you could say, a necessity, as it was somewhere they could both retreat from the increasingly stressful weeks at the Court, and George, who had not long ago recovered from a nervous breakdown, found a real sense of peace there. In fact this proved to be doubly necessary as a month or so before William was born he suffered a heart attack and, although this was not life-threatening, he was told to take complete rest and went into a peaceful period of semi-retirement at Andrews' Farm. So Peter and I would be invited down for weekends, and walk in the countryside, sit in the garden, eat in the kitchen. I have a clear vision of standing outside the farm with my father patting me gently on my growing bump and saying softly, 'Little mother!'.

One of the best things about being pregnant was that I ended up having a companion during the last few months of the process. This was my oldest and dearest friend Catherine Turner. She and I had not seen so much of each other in recent years. She had gone to Oxford to read Modern Languages, and I had plunged into drama school and boyfriends. We had never lost touch, but in the past year had not met at all because she had gone for a year abroad and had taken it in Moscow, Russian being one of her languages. While she was there, she had fallen in love with an American academic and had come back to England pregnant: her baby was due just two weeks before mine. However, pregnant she may have been but married she was not. In fact Dan Mulholland, the baby's father, was married to somebody else.

Mark and Peggy Turner were outraged. She could not, they told her, stay in their house while she was pregnant — what would the neighbours think? She must find somewhere else to live and, they insisted, she must have the baby adopted after it was born. This Catherine had no intention of doing since she had become pregnant quite deliberately, taking the view that if she had lost Dan she would at least have something to remember him by. This attitude did not help her relations with her parents, who booked her into a repressive home for unmarried mothers for the final weeks of her pregnancy and arranged for her to stay as a paying guest and general dogsbody with an acquaintance of theirs who, by chance, happened to live just round the corner from Lower Mall.

Of course she came to visit my mother, and Sophie was horrified to hear what her parents had done. So before much time had passed, Catherine had moved in to Lower Mall, where she would stay until just before her baby was born. For me this was great. Peter and I were living on our tiny, rather cramped but very pretty houseboat, the HB Patriarch, but as Peter was at work all day I spent most of my time at Lower Mall anyway, and now I had someone to talk to about the pleasures and displeasures of pregnancy, someone to knit with, a friend and companion. Although there was an obvious discrepancy between our two situations, Catherine was as cheerful and determined as circumstances allowed and we managed to have an enormous amount of fun. The best thing, perhaps, was discovering that we had (and still have) the kind of friendship that persists through long absences and can constantly reinvent itself and adapt to changing circumstances.

Fortunately this story had a happy ending. When Mark and Peggy visited Catherine after her daughter Anna was born they fell immediately in love with the baby. Adoption was now out of the question — Anna had to stay. So they bought Cathy a house in Camden Town, which my mother helped her to furnish, and before long Dan astonished everyone by turning up, getting

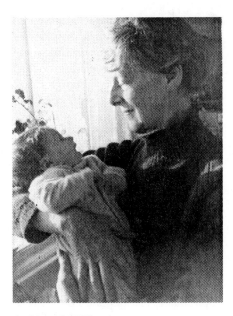

*Sophie with William*

divorced, marrying Catherine and taking her off to live with him in America.

Soon after Anna was born it was my turn. My due date, 11 November, came and went and nothing happened. I spent the weekend making Christmas puddings and feeling impatient and frustrated. Pregnancy is bearable when you have days to cross off on the calendar but once that comes to an end time seems to pass with appalling slowness. I remembered that someone had told me that if you took castor oil it could bring on your labour, so I tried it, and sure enough in the early hours of 14 November I started to have contractions. I had a long and tiring day of it, but finally, at ten thirty that night, William appeared. There was a momentary panic when he was born as he was not breathing, but the doctor put a tiny mask over his face and sucked mechanically until he started. Once he got going he was an excellent baby, healthy and happy. He had a mass of black hair which lay as if rather neatly brushed forward on his forehead, and everyone said he looked like one of the Beatles.

# 12

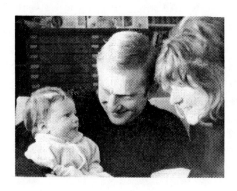

*William being adored by his parents*

Being a mother turned out to be all right. I had been pretty dubious about it merely because I had never in my entire life even so much as held a baby in my arms before William was born, apart from one occasion at a party when I had been handed one which began to cry straight away and got hastily handed back to where it belonged. And here I was with one of my own. I found out that within a day or two you know exactly what to do. The process was made easier by the fact that I loved William so much. A rather selfish and self-absorbed sort of person, I was completely unprepared for the kind of unconditional love that seemed to sweep me off my feet and, incidentally, slowly made me realise just how much feeling was missing from my relationship with Peter. William was a delightful baby, admired by passing old ladies as well as loved by the family. He learned to laugh very quickly and seemed to enjoy doing it a lot, sitting in his pram outside shops chuckling away at private jokes of his own.

Sophie absolutely adored him, and he adored her. In fact she was happy to take him off for the day and play with him endlessly, which was good for me as I was able to have a bit of necessary breathing-space. I took him out myself a good deal: often Cathy and I would meet in Highgate and take our babies for walks in the cemetery. Our childish ability to giggle seemed as much in evidence as ever and we had a lot of fun peering into mausoleums to see if we could see any bodies, or reading the writing on the tombstones and making up songs about them. 'Seventy-seven and never forgotten', for example, became a sort of calypso: 'He was seventy-seven and we'll never forget him/ Though the grass may grow and the dew may wet him'. Extremely silly for a couple of young adults, but it did us good. Cathy was very unsure about what her future was going to be, and I was, increasingly, aware that I was not happy with Peter. I was a long way from making any kind of decision at this stage, however. I may not have felt the right things for Peter but I did like being married, in the sense that I enjoyed life as part of a couple, and did not even consider for a moment the possibility of going back to a single life.

Soon after William was born Peter was offered a chance to go and work in the South of France, something I was only too delighted for him to do as I could go along as well — another overseas adventure. The place we were to go was called Ramatuelle, and it was a hill village in the bay overlooking St Tropez. I had been to this part of the world before, on the holiday to Gassin with my mother, Cathy and Claire. So I knew how beautiful the area was and encouraged Peter to take the chance to go. He had been increasingly discontented with his furniture designing, so he resigned from the job and decided he would be able to support us being free-lance.

The trip to Ramatuelle was arranged by a friend of Peter's by the name of Peter Crofton-Sleigh, a tall, thin, grizzled, bearded man with a public-school accent who made his living doing up people's houses. Peter had got to know him at a cafe called The Troubadour in Earls Court. The house they were going to do up belonged to a daughter of Augustus John, although she used it only occasionally. So a few days after Christmas, William, now exactly six weeks old, and I got onto a plane and flew to Nice. The two Peters had set off earlier in Peter Crofton-Sleigh's disreputable jeep, and after William and I had spent a night in a rather nice hotel the jeep appeared at the door and we were whisked off down the Grand Corniche. It was not exactly warm, but the sky was clear pale blue, the sun bright and pale yellow, and my spirits rose hugely. At St Tropez we turned right, up a twisting road through woods which promised to be full of mimosa, and finally turned into the square at Ramatuelle.

I fell completely in love with the town straight away. It was an ancient stone construction, all built in a spiral — the tiny internal lanes just twisted round and round until they reached the middle. A consequence of the way it was built was that all the houses overlapped each other. In ours, for example, you went in through the front door, up a flight of stairs, and by the time you got to the living room you were over the top of the ground floor of the house next door. Another fight of stairs led you to the bedrooms, which were similarly displaced, so that in a sense everyone was living on top of or underneath their neighbours. Since the walls and floors were so thick, though, this hardly seemed to matter.

The job of the two Peters was, essentially, to pull the whole place apart and put it back together again. This would take about three months. My job, meanwhile, was to look after William, cook, and clean. Cleaning was, alas, not my forte. I had hardly ever cleaned the boat — in fact my mother had been in the habit of coming round there once a week to wash up and put things away for me. Peter Crofton-Sleigh thought that cleaning was woman's work and said so very frequently, which made me absolutely furious, so that we used to have huge rows about it. Cooking, on the other hand, I enjoyed a lot. I discovered that there were, in the bookshelf, a whole collection of French recipe books by chefs with famous names like Escoffier, and I made it my business to experiment with the recipes. The village had a small supermarket where I would go and buy the ingredients for the exciting meals that appeared on the table every night. I never had the nerve, or even the desire, to buy from the *chasseur*, who walked through the village several times a week with a long wooden pole over his shoulder from which hung tiny dead birds which he sold to the locals. If they were not bought warm from the gun, they ended up plucked and brown in the deep-freeze of the supermarket.

I cooked and cooked, and the two Peters were hugely appreciative of the results, but I never thought about how much I was spending on the food. Then one day Peter Crofton-Sleigh discovered how far I had exceeded the budget and there was another huge row. Repentant, I promised to cut down but I was not very good at economising and the trouble was that there was little for me to do besides cook. William was a good baby — I carried him around in a little blue fabric sling so that he was tucked into my side, and one day an old lady at a market caught sight of him there and said he was '*exactement comme un petit oiseau*'. I found how much I enjoyed talking French, and amazed the two Peters one day when a man came to the door on business and I rattled away at him like a native. The only problem was that my accent was rather in advance of my comprehension and my vocabulary so I was constantly being taken for a more fluent speaker than I actually was.

As time went on the weather started to improve and soon it was quite warm. Then I would put William in his pram and we would go for long walks down the hillside and among the fields of the surrounding countryside, looking longingly at little stone farmhouses and exchanging polite greetings with rather surprised locals. Once a week, on a Friday evening, we went to the cafe in the square and made a reverse-charge call to Sophie back in England, and I wrote long letters to both my parents with drawings and plans of the village and stories of its history.

Our stay there would have been idyllic apart from the ideological differences between me and Peter Crofton-Sleigh. Although I had never heard of feminism I could not subscribe to his view that women's place was in the kitchen. After all, this had not been my experience: my mother had always worked and her job had always seemed as important as my father's so this seemed to me to be a normal state of affairs. I did try out one of his recommendations, though. William had one time of day — about six in the evening — when he had a burst of crying for an hour or so. I was in the habit of going and picking him up, carrying him around and jiggling him about until he finally stopped. But Peter Crofton-Sleigh said that this was bad for him, that he would be spoiled. He suggested we just left him to cry, and said that if we did he would soon learn to stop. So we decided to try it. At six o'clock the tiny cries began, getting louder and more frantic by the minute. Peter Key and I sat, clutching each other, pale and rigid, as we tried to ignore them. But we were just not cut out for it. I stood it for about twenty minutes and then I cracked, and would never try it again. It could not be right, I thought, so much pain on both sides.

It was early April by the time the work was finished, and the countryside was warm and golden, smelling of wild thyme, with mimosa blossom appearing on the trees. I took to sunbathing on the flat roof of the house and started to turn a rather pinky sort of brown. But now we had to go home. This time it was decided that I would travel back in the jeep. Peter Crofton-Sleigh wanted to do the whole journey in one, driving fast, to get to Calais in about twenty-four hours. This proved to be a little over-optimistic. The two Peters sat in the front, taking turns to drive, and William and I were in the back, rattling and bumping, catching a bit of sleep when we were able to. After a miserable day and night we were still many hours from Calais and decided to stop in a cafe for some lunch. By now the weather was dark, cold and rainy. William was still wearing the same clothes I had put on him when we left — I had just managed to change his nappies but anything else was impractical. As we sat huddled and exhausted at a table waiting for our food, I noticed a family of respectable middle-class French persons at the next table looking at us in open horror and amazement. We must have been a travel-stained and peculiar-looking bunch — Peter Crofton-Sleigh, with his long beard and many knitted scarves was particularly striking. But it was William who was attracting the most attention — his white Babygro was grey to the point of blackness. A large French child gazed at him for a while and then turned to her mother and said loudly, pointing at him, 'Comme il est sale!', which made me feel rather ashamed.

So back to England it was, and back to life on the houseboat. Peter was back to work and I was back to being a rather reluctant housewife and mother. Luckily Sophie continued to demand time with William and I was able to have driving lessons, after which I rather triumphantly passed my test first time and bought an ancient and wonderful car. It was called a Wolsely 12 and it was black and shiny with a silver-capped bonnet —the kind of car you see the police driving in films from the 1940s. It sat in the road across from the moorings until one night it got completely destroyed in rather a dramatic way. A drunk in a red sports car came whizzing round the corner and smashed into a car which was three behind mine with such force that all the cars in the road concertinaed into each other. We came out in the morning to find another car had inserted itself into the Wolsely and was sitting with its front wheels resting on my dashboard.

This was exciting, but in general life on the boat was more and more boring. It was easier when William was tiny and happy to lie in his carrycot chortling away to himself, as I could read and watch television and cook. But soon he became very active. By the time he was seven months old he was crawling, and this made life increasingly difficult. He crawled in a most unusual way, on his hands and feet rather than his knees, so that it was like having a small dog in the room, racing around at terrific speed. Now it became quite impossible to do anything as he had to be watched every minute of the time, and I began to go completely mad with the boredom of it all. The boat was tiny and he would go round and round in this tiny space, pulling everything apart. Being on the river with a tiny active child was also rather scary as the Thames, brown and glutinous, was only a few feet away, slapping and slopping against the side of the boat. This became a real worry. He was far too little to be taught not to go near the water, and I was exhausted with constantly restraining him.

Luckily, soon after his first birthday, Sophie came up with a suggestion.

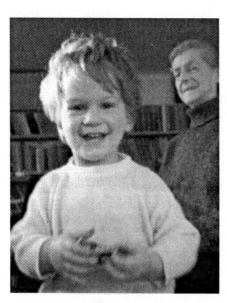

*Sophie with William aged about one*

Peter could do a conversion at Lower Mall, build some extra rooms out into the garden and convert the strange, long, gloomy extension into two separate bedrooms. Then we could sell the boat and move back in. This seemed liked the best idea in the world — company for me, company for Sophie. And so began a long and grubby summer, with dust and woodshavings everywhere, but before too long the place was finished and I was living back at Lower Mall again. By the time we moved in, William had stopped being a baby and become a fine, strong, handsome little boy, with his father's shapely physique, blue eyes, and hair that was no longer black but a sort of ash blond. He loved to play with Peter's woodworking tools, and tried endlessly to help with the work on the house. Also he loved to draw, presumably a result of hours spent sitting beside my mother at the kitchen table watching her doing her designs.

While all this was going on, my father was once again getting driven into the ground by the hard work of running the Court. He may have backed off from being much of a father to me, but he certainly was experiencing all the traditional problems of fatherhood with the assistant artistic directors at the Court. He continued to try and delegate responsibility but as always no one was fully prepared to take it on. On top of all this he was constantly having to intervene in squabbles between two of his assistant directors, Lindsay Anderson and Anthony Page, squabbles which culminated in Lindsay's resignation and more work devolving onto George himself. As well as his work for the ESC he had directed Beckett's *Play* at the National Theatre. This was due to move into a new building and George got involved with the planning, working closely with the architect Denis Lasdun. Tired and disheartened, despite the huge success of John Osborne's latest play *Inadmissible Evidence*, he decided to resign from the ESC and wrote a letter to the Council informing them of the fact.

A few months later his resignation was made public at a lunch for the critics at the Savoy Hotel. His retirement speech summed up how fundamentally necessary this move to withdraw had come to seem:

*When a man comes to feel he is part of the fixtures and fittings, it is time he left. I am deeply tired. The weight of this edifice has driven me into the ground, like poor Winnie in Beckett's Happy Days. I should have passed the job on years ago. I am getting out just in time.*

He may have wanted to give up the Court, but he was not planning to sit back and do nothing. He had been offered a job which he very much wanted to do: directing the running of a new Arts Centre which was being planned and built at Sussex University. The job, which meant involving young people in the creative life of the university and local community, seemed to be ideal for him: less taxing than the Court, but sufficiently engaging of his ideals and aspirations to keep him contentedly at work until the age when he could properly retire.

Shortly before his appointment was confirmed, George met with the university's Vice Chancellor, Sir John Fulton, and various other notables. Wanting to have his appointment made with full clarity as to the facts of his life, he asked to make a statement. He wanted them to know that he was not prepared to participate in organised religion of any description, and that he was living with a woman who was not his wife. Honest though he had been, I think he was not prepared for the response, which came by letter shortly afterwards. Fulton wrote to say that, while the religious issue was not a problem, they were unable to offer him the post because of his openness about his relationship with Jocelyn. As he discovered later, a blind eye would have been turned to this if he had kept silent, but could not now that he had announced it so publicly. Shocked, he decided to take an appointment that had been offered him in Brazil, running the Theatre Conservatory in Rio. He and Jocelyn would be able to live there in peace. Meanwhile he had some months left to work out his contract at the Court.

As for me, I had embarked on a challenging little task of my own: a tremendous diet. I had put on weight during the pregnancy and found to my shame that I had crept back to my boarding-school size and that the lovely clothes I had imagined wearing once William was born were simply not a possibility. So I found a doctor, a friend of Peter Key's called Geoffrey Gray, who had a practice in Chelsea and who reckoned he had a miracle cure for fatness. You had to go and see him every day and he would give you an injection of some mystery substance, reputed to be derived from some unmentionable part of a cow. Then you would eat a very limited diet and behold! You would lose weight. Naturally I have realised since that you would lose weight anyway from following his diet, which consisted mainly of a tiny slice of meat and a couple of small heaps of vegetables twice a day, but even if the injections were a placebo they were a help. Because you

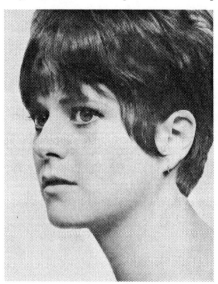

had to pay Geoffrey and have them every day you felt — or I certainly did — under an obligation to do the job properly. And so I did. After one course I had lost a stone, and a second course a few months later left me absolutely sylphlike, for the first time within my memory.

No one who has not been distinctly plump for almost all their lives will be able to understand what effect this had on me. Suddenly I could look at myself in the mirror and be really delighted with what I saw. And I played it up to the full. A wonderful shop called Biba had just opened in Kensington: the clothes seemed to me to be perfect

*After my great diet*

and were not at all expensive, and I became one of their best customers. I bought a patterned trouser suit, newly fashionable mini-dresses, skinny skirts and tops. I had my hair carefully arranged in a cascade of curls on top of my head, I wore pale lipstick and much black kohl around my eyes.

I loved myself, and, what's more, everyone seemed to love me. And, I'm sorry to say, I played that up to the full as well. The kissing at parties, which had ground to a halt with the marriage and the pregnancy, started up again with a vengeance. Often Peter was present, but he never said a word. This should have made me feel even guiltier, but in fact I hardly felt guilty at all. I fell madly in love with Peter O'Toole, an old friend of Peter's, though all he did was flirt with me at a party. I spent another party, at Rossetti Studios, locked in the arms of Jenny Lousada's boyfriend, a handsome actor called Drewe Henley, and an evening in a house in Hammersmith Terrace passionately embracing John Hurt in the presence of not only Peter but also of John's wife, my friend Annette. I behaved outrageously with Stephen Frears, an up-and-coming young director, and with my old friend David Warner, both of them working at the time on a film called *Morgan: A Suitable Case for Treatment*.

The summer of my great diet, my mother was asked to design a production of Pinero's *Trelawny of the 'Wells'* at the new Chichester Festival Theatre. She asked me if I would like to come down and stay in the house she had rented, in the grand seaside town West Wickham, and off I went down there for six weeks taking eighteen-month-old William. We had a great time and Sophie did some beautiful costumes of just the lush Victorian kind that she always designed so well. We had a real sense of being on holiday and managed some hugely enjoyable days out and some great giggles together. William was a joy. He was learning to speak at a frightening rate — I tried to make a list of all the words he knew but had to give up, as there were too many new ones every day. He also succeeded in destroying not only the car headlights but also the expensive dining-room table in the rented house by some judicious use of his little toy hammer. At Chichester I also managed to behave outrageously yet again with an ugly but attractive actor by the name of Ron Pember.

Clearly this couldn't go on indefinitely. I remember vividly a painful occasion during our stay down there when Peter turned up, having not seen me for weeks, and I could not raise the faintest enthusiasm for his presence, never mind for what he wanted to do in bed. In fact since I had had William I had found that I simply did not fancy Peter any more, and this, obviously, caused big problems. Back in London, I had started living an increasingly separate life, spending less and less time with Peter and more and more with Georgina, my friend from LAMDA, and the new and exciting circle of friends she had acquired.

Despite studying it for two years, Georgina had never actually gone into stage management. She did work at the Royal Court for a while, helping Keith Johnstone (with whom she was briefly involved) to set up a scheme for sixth-formers to visit the theatre and take part in workshops run by Keith, but when the scheme and the relationship came to an end she had managed to take up with a Jamaican trumpet player called Gary. Tall, skinny and charming, Gary was also, it is sad to record, something of a psychopath and would from time to time subject her to mental and physical abuse. The two of them were living in a basement flat at the top of Baker Street that belonged to Georgina's father, and Gary was anxious to make his name in the world of music. So Georgina, who had come into a small inheritance at twenty-one, agreed to help him form a band and to be its manager.

Musicians had to be recruited, and Gary had contacts, obviously. Soon there was a band, called The Sidewinders, made up of a mixture of black and white musicians, who played a kind of mix of jazz and blues in various venues in and around London. Before he moved to London, Gary had lived in Guildford, and one of the musicians he recruited came from there. He was the drummer, and his name was Alan Mennie, though everyone always called him by his nickname, which was Min. I didn't take much notice of him at first, as he was rather quiet, though I could see he was quite beautiful, tall and slender, with long auburn hair and large, soulful eyes.

Life at the flat was pretty chaotic, as most of the band seemed to sleep there on most nights. During the day when they were not playing they would sit around listening to music and smoking pot. I soon enjoyed doing the same things, and would go with them on their gigs as well, to places like Eel Pie Island, where they would be supporting more successful people like Long John Baldry.

The problem was that nobody had any money, and the gigs were too poorly paid to support them all. Then Georgina found a useful source of income. On the radio there was a weekly phone-in programme run by a disc jockey called Jimmy Young. Starting at ten at night and continuing until two, it was named, rather unimaginatively, Through till Two. People could call the BBC all through this four-hour period and ask for records to be played, and a large number of people was needed to answer the phones. So the whole band, apart from Gary for some reason, started to work there, and as I did everything they did I started to work there too. For the relatively small number of hours involved the pay was quite good, perhaps as much as £10 for two nights' work. This was not as essential for me as it was for the band, who used it to pay the rent — I used it to buy more clothes at Biba and have my hair done.

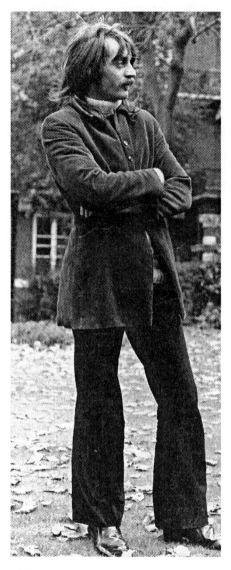

*Min*

So twice every week we all trundled off to Langham Place and sat by our telephones saying endlessly 'Through till Two!', and writing down the requests on little slips of paper which were somehow selected and passed through to Jimmy Young who then put the records on. It was during our first weeks at Langham Place that I suddenly became aware of Min in a powerful and dangerous way. It began, I remember, with him coming towards me on the pavement outside the BBC, taking my hand and lifting it to his mouth, gazing into my eyes as he did so. I felt as if my heart did actually turn over, though I suppose it can't have done really. Soon we were friends and very soon after that it was clear that we were falling in love.

Frequently silent in mixed company, Min was communicative to me. He told me all about his disastrous marriage — at art-school aged eighteen, to his pregnant girl-friend — his two little boys, in Surrey with their mother and rarely seen, and his parents, kind and simple folk who lived in a little council house in Guildford. We turned out to be almost the same age — at just twenty-three he was six months older than I was. One day he came round to Lower Mall and I opened the door to him with William perched on my hip and Min was completely bowled over by him: 'What a fantastic kid!'. He started to write me intense, passionate love letters. I was completely swept away by it all. Nothing in the world seemed to matter except the two of us and our feeling for each other.

It was impossible for us not to become lovers, and indeed it seemed like the most right and natural thing in the world. Just as impossible was not to spend all our time together. So when I was not at Baker Street Min was at Lower Mall. My mother liked him enormously, as did Percy, who appreciated his capacity for drinking whisky. Peter liked him rather less. Nobody, though, seemed to notice what was going on, or, more likely, nobody wanted to notice. We became more and more outrageous: on one rather shameful occasion we went downstairs and made love on my bed while Sophie and Peter were upstairs in the sitting room with William.

Obviously this could not go on for ever. It began in the summer, and by the end of October Sophie clearly had become rather worried. One day she said to me, rather more irritated than anything else, 'You seem to spend *all* your time with Min!'.

> *I'm in love with him,* I said, probably rather relieved to get it into the open.
> *Are you having an affair?*
> *Yes, we are.*

Poor Sophie — the second time she had confronted me with such a question, and the second time I had given her a dusty answer. The first time, with Chris, everyone seemed to accept it all pretty quickly and it blew over fast. This time was a much more painful occasion. Both she and Peter, who had to be told straight away, were deeply upset and deeply angry.

# 13

Obviously things could not go on as they had been now that my relationship with Min was out in the open. My mother and Peter confronted me with an ultimatum. I had to make a choice. If I wanted to be with Min I must leave Lower Mall, and leave William — they would take care of him. If I wanted William I must give up Min. They had no legal right to make this threat, but none of us was thinking very clearly and it seemed pretty serious to me. Evidently, as even I was aware, it was designed to bring me to my senses, but all I could see was that I could not give up either of them.

Min said he would take me away for a few days to think. He had an uncle who was a coastguard at St David's, the most westerly part of Wales, and the next day the two of us set off in my tiny little Fiat 600, rattling down the main roads on a nine-hour journey. Min was gentle and loving, and I — I was completely shell-shocked. Min's uncle was kind, St David's was stunningly beautiful, and we spent four days there, just walking on the cliffs and on the empty sandy beaches. A photo taken there shows me looking strained and deeply unhappy. Clearly I could not live without William.

Luckily when we got back to Lower Mall everyone had calmed down a bit and Sophie and Peter had realised that the thing was not workable. Apart from anything else both of them were working and could not possibly manage to look after William. So after a tense conference a plan was made. I would move in with Min, who had a flat in Westbourne Grove, but every day I would come to Lower Mall early in the morning, get William up, spend the day with him and leave again after I had put him to bed. It was not a very satisfactory arrangement, but we played it that way for about six weeks, and then my mother found a flat for the three of us to move into. It was in Fulham, opposite St Stephen's Hospital, and Min and I and William moved in there in December.

And so was played out my biggest personal drama so far. In a sense I was sorry that I had not behaved very well towards Peter and had upset my mother, but all in all I was glad, as being with Min made me spectacularly happy. Peter behaved with great dignity, and we managed to stay (and have remained) good friends. I suppose you could say that marrying him in the first place, given my ambivalent feelings, was the biggest mistake, but if I had not I would not have had William, to whom he remained the best of

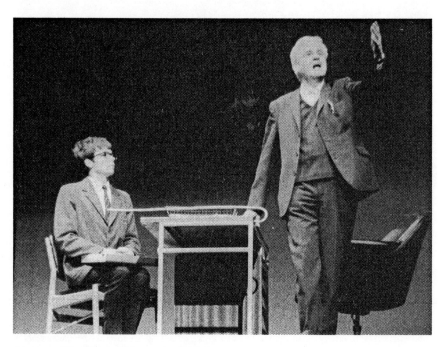

*George with Richard James in* Miniatures

fathers even though mostly in absentia.

And what of my own father? Although he had seemed well and happy in the early part of this year, and gave a superb comic performance in Donald Howarth's Sunday night production of David Cregan's *Miniatures,* he had decided to resign from the English Stage Company, and was working out the last few months of his contract. Not surprisingly, he was getting exhausted again. In August, Peter and I had been invited to spend the weekend at Andrews' Farm, and had turned up on Friday evening. Jocelyn was on her own at the farm as my father was playing at the Court, and would be for another week. The play he was in was John Osborne's extraordinary and powerful black comedy of the homosexual underworld in late nineteenth-century Austria, *A Patriot for Me.* John had written a part especially for him, the transvestite homosexual Baron von Epp, and George played the entire show dressed like Queen Alexandra in a tiara, a choker, evening-dress and pearls. It was one of his most memorable performances. On the Saturday of our weekend in Hampshire, he was due to play two shows and to come down to Andrews' after the evening performance.

At the matinee were some very special visitors. They were members of the Berliner Ensemble, including my father's good friend Helene Weigel, the widow of Brecht. Naturally there was a party between the shows, and then another performance to give. George was not feeling well, and had some warning pains in his chest, but he laced on his corset and went ahead with the show.

Meanwhile, Peter and I had put William to bed and were having supper with Jocelyn in the farmhouse when someone tapped loudly on the window. It was an employee of the post-office — Andrews' was not on the telephone, and he had come across the fields to deliver an urgent telegram. My father had had a serious heart attack and had been rushed to St

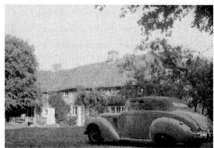

*George's Alvis outside Andrew's Farm*

George's Hospital. Jocelyn dropped everything, got into her car and raced to London, leaving us to lock the place up and follow next morning.

Unpleasant and uncomfortable though the ward was, and awful though it was for Jocelyn to be refused entrance initially, since for some reason my father's doctor, John Henderson, had put my mother's name down as next-of-kin, George seemed as if he was going to get better. A week later John Osborne announced as much to the audience attending the last night of *Patriot*, and we all started to feel confident that he would soon be back on his feet. But then the real blow struck. About ten days after the heart attack my father suffered a massive stroke, which paralysed him down the left side of his body, and he was not expected to recover.

Jocelyn and Tony Richardson, believing the hospital had given him up for good, managed to see a private specialist and a drug called propranolol was prescribed. The doctor told them honestly that there was a fifty per cent chance of this killing him, but the other alternative seemed so desperate that they decided to go ahead. Luckily the drug did appear to reverse some of the damage and before long he was able to see visitors, though clearly he was depressed and angry at the continuing paralysis and the fact that he could only speak with difficulty using one side of his mouth.

It must have been before this drug was administered that I was allowed to visit him for the first time after his stroke. He was by this time in a small side ward, by himself. It was a huge shock to see him like this: skin and bone, in hospital nightwear, on a battered iron bed. The ward sister ushered me in and I sat on a chair beside him and took his hand. Did he know who I was? Barely and intermittently perhaps he did, but he was only half-conscious and when he did seem to be awake and looking around him he was not at all sure where he was, taking me sometimes for my mother and sometimes for nurses in India and Burma. He talked and talked, or muttered and mumbled, and I soon gave up trying to respond and just sat there, shocked but unable to move, for at least an hour. Then the sister came in and registered surprise at finding me still there, as she had only meant for me to stay ten minutes.

When he had recovered sufficiently, he was briefly moved to the Middlesex Hospital, and I went to see him there after the turmoil of leaving Peter. He was much better by now, though still partly paralysed, and was sitting up in bed, thin and weak, his eyes ringed with brown. 'Lovely to see you, my darling', he said, and I really felt that this was true. He was not up to much conversation, and part of the time we sat there in silence, but soon he turned to me and said, 'I hear you've got yourself a new man'. 'Yes,' I said.

*And is he making you happy?*
*Yes, very happy.*
*I'm really glad.*

I wanted him to meet Min, and soon after this visit the opportunity came. George was discharged from hospital in early November and went home to Rossetti Studios. Jocelyn had set the place up to meet his needs and he was able to sit up during the day either in bed or in a wheelchair and talk to friends. On his birthday, 20 November, there was a party and I took Min along. With all the people there they were not able to do more than just say hello, but I was glad to have had the chance to introduce them and hoped that they might get to know each other better in the future.

But what kind of future would there be for George? Seeing him there in his wheelchair it was impossible not to realise that inside that semi-useless body was a mind, as quick and alert as ever, which was wild with frustration and disappointment at being trapped inside, unable to use the energy and activity to which it was so accustomed. I was unavoidably reminded of two parts he had played, two awful previsions of his present state: the dying actor in the Chekhov television play, and above all Hamm in *Endgame*, blind and paralysed, abusing God – 'the bastard, he doesn't exist'.

After the party I visited him quite often, taking William, now two, along with me. To tell the truth it was nice just to be able to drop in, to find him always at home. I would tell him what I was up to — mostly house hunting, as Min and I had only a limited tenancy in the flat we were in — and William would chatter away, as two-year-olds do, perched on the end of the bed. And so, I suppose, things might have gone on indefinitely. George called in Christine Smith, his wonderful loyal secretary from the Court, and began to dictate the autobiography that had been commissioned by Faber. This is part of what he wrote:

*I was not strictly after a popular theatre a la Joan Littlewood-Roger Planchon, but a theatre that would be part of the intellectual life of the country. In this respect I consider I utterly failed. I feel I have the right to talk in this proprietary was about the English Stage Company, to which I gave nine years of my life and nearly died in the tenth. I was convinced the way to achieve my objective was to get writers, writers of serious pretensions, back into the theatre. This I set out to do. I wanted to change the attitude of the public towards the theatre. All I did was to change the attitude of the theatre towards the public....*

*Peter Hall has called the theatre a brothel. I don't agree. For me it is a temple of ideas, and ideas so well expressed it may be called art. So always look for the quality of the writing above what is being said. This is how to choose a theatre to write in and if you can't find one you like, start your own. A theatre must have a recognisable attitude. It will have one whether it likes it or not.*

So that was keeping his mind alert. A physiotherapist came to help him with exercises designed to bring his body back to something resembling normal use. But before this object was achieved, on 29 January 1966, George had another heart attack and died. He was just fifty-five years old.

I suppose such an outcome had always been a possibility, but it was no less of a shock for that. In fact it was so much of a shock that it was hard to take it in. The only positive thing you could say about it was that at least he died at home, in the arms of the person that he loved, rather than in one of the grim hospital wards where his life had been under such severe threat earlier. It was terrible for Jocelyn, who had endured so many months of fear and uncertainty and who seemed for a while as if she had got him back. But it was terrible for my mother, too, and in a sense it was almost harder for her since she did not have the official position of the widow. To me she never spoke of how she felt — she always kept her deepest feelings to herself. But seeing her in the days after his death, tightly controlled and determined to go on, one had the sense of being with someone who had sustained a mortal wound.

A couple of days after George's death I had a message from Jocelyn's son Julian Lousada. He wanted to come and talk to me urgently. We met at Lower Mall. Julian seemed awkward and embarrassed, but he came to the point quickly. 'George does not seem to have made a will, which means everything will go to you, and poor Mummy will be destitute. Will you consider sharing half of what you are going to get?'

But what was there to inherit? Until very recently the answer would have been absolutely nothing. George's salary at the Court was laughably small, by his own choice, and neither of my parents ever had any savings. Lower Mall was my mother's house and he had left, when he left, with nothing but his clothes and his books. However, now there was something — in fact there was seventeen thousand pounds, no mean sum in 1966. This was the money that had come from the film of *Tom Jones*. My father, like many of the actors in the film, had accepted a pay deal that involved a minimal payment at the time of filming and a percentage of the profits, if there were any. The profits were huge and so, at the time of his death, George had money for the first time in his life.

I could see no reason why I should not give half to Jocelyn and I told Julian to contact me again in a few days to talk more about it. But then before I could call him, he called me again. A will had turned up, in, of all places, the solicitors' offices of Jocelyn's ex-husband, Anthony Lousada. And the will said that everything he possessed should go to Jocelyn. So that was the end of that short-lived saga, at least as far as the negotiations went. For my own feelings it was not the end. All my old sense of rejection, which had been in retreat over the past few months of closeness to George, was revived by the feeling that he had cut me out of his life. Carefully it was explained to me that the will had been made at the request of Anthony Lousada himself, who had refused to give Jocelyn custody of the children unless my father willed everything to her. Since this all happened before the *Tom Jones* money appeared, George must have felt it was pretty much of an academic exercise. And he was also aware that I would be inheriting my mother's property, including Lower Mall, at some stage. All of this seemed eminently sensible, but it did not take away the hurt. Indeed, twenty years later, in the course of researching an obscure eighteenth-century poet, I visited the wills department of Somerset House. Failing Akenside's will, I decided to look at my father's, and discovered that, even after so much time, seeing it in black and white still had power to cause me intense pain. But he did not mean it like that.

However little I had initially managed to take in the fact of my father's death, it was brought home to me by the funeral. This was for me, and others too, I think, an unusually grim and depressing affair. It took place in the early days of February, on a dark, cold day. Rain poured on us all as we shuffled through the doors of the chapel at Golders Green Crematorium. It seemed a huge and cavernous place, full of distinguished persons come to mourn George. The remaining Boys, Glen and Michel, were there and many other friends from the olden days, and all the new friends, the writers, directors and actors from the Court. There was a certain amount of awkwardness for some people, friends of both my mother and of Jocelyn, who found it difficult to know which side of the chapel to sit — seating seeming naturally to have divided itself between supporters of the two women in his life. My mother sat between Peter Gill and Percy, both of whom were in floods of tears while she remained grim but determinedly dry-eyed.

I found the service peculiar and unsatisfying. Jocelyn had felt, probably quite rightly, that as a declared atheist George would not have wanted a religious service, and so the music was resolutely secular: Thelonious Monk was played as the coffin trundled in, and Benjamin Britten at the end. Probably he would have been happy with this, but it did not suit my manqué Catholicism. I wanted prayers and anthems and chanting and wafting incense, though George certainly would have hated the thought of all this. Anyway, soon it was over and we all went off to get on with the rest of our lives as best we could.

For me, that meant trying to adjust to living with Min. Not that being with him did not make me happy. In a purely personal sense I had a sense of rightness that I had never experienced before. But from a more practical angle there were evident problems, the chief of which was money. The only source of income we had was a tiny allowance that my mother had set up for me when I got married, a typically generous gesture and one she could ill afford. But this was not really enough to live on. From Peter I got nothing. He had taken off to Greece shortly after we broke up, on a protracted holiday designed to heal his wounds, and though he came back a few months later with not one but two women in tow, one of whom he eventually married, I did not then nor indeed in the future feel right about asking him for money even to support William.

So money was a definite worry. Georgina's band suddenly fell apart at this point, Gary having finally departed, and so Min had no visible means of support. When I tried to suggest that he might get a job to help with the situation, he retired to bed and refused to speak. When I finally managed to get him to explain, he said his wife had nagged him endlessly about working to support her and the boys and that he refused to be drawn into a similar state of affairs. He also would not sign on as he was trying to keep a low profile as far as officialdom was concerned: his wife wanted him to pay maintenance for the children and he refused on the grounds that she was being supported in some comfort by her wealthy parents. His hope seemed to be that if he kept himself out of sight for long enough he would simply disappear from the record altogether. He would have considered earning money as a musician, but he lacked contacts and no one seemed prepared to offer him any work.

I was fairly desperate about all this, and also trying to look after a two-year-old. Soon the housing situation caught up with us too. The Fulham flat we had been living in belonged to a friend of my mother's but this was understood to be a limited agreement. It came to an even sharper close one day when our landlady visited us and discovered our attempts to bring the decor into the 1960s. We had not asked her permission before painting the bathroom black with red abstract images floating on the walls, and she, appalled, asked us to find another place to live as soon as possible.

So now I was out every day house hunting. I tried to get Min to help me, but he retired to bed again. I soon found that the usual sources, agents and the *Evening Standard*, were a waste of time, as all the flats were either horrible or had gone before I got there. Every morning I would get William dressed and into his pushchair and set off to pound the streets. It seemed like a good idea to stay within striking distance of Lower Mall as we still spent a great deal of time there when Sophie was not too busy to see us. She was working hard as usual, designing a film for Roman Polanski, but we always spent weekends with her. She and William had a great relationship and she naturally wanted to see as much of him as possible, having been part of his life for so long.

Because of wanting to stay close to my mother, I started to look at flats in Putney. It was within walking distance of Hammersmith, along the very pretty towpath, and seemed to have a lot of large Victorian apartment blocks, which looked as if they would be worth investigating. This was the first time I had ever done any house hunting and I found it a depressing business. William and I would trawl the streets and when we saw a likely looking building we would go to the porter's office to see if there were any empty flats. But everywhere we went we met a blank wall.

I quickly became very despondent. Then one day I was trying what was virtually my last hope, a small block called University Mansions, close to the river in Lower Richmond Road. The porter was brusque and unhelpful as usual, and I turned miserably away down the road, pushing the pushchair towards Putney Bridge and wondering what on earth to do next. Suddenly I was tapped on the shoulder by a large and kindly looking man. He was an actor, as it turned out, and indeed quite an actor-laddie sort of person, in a large camel-coloured overcoat with a fur collar. He had overheard my conversation with the porter and thought he could help. He was about to move out of a top floor flat in the block but had not yet told the management, and he offered to let me move in first and square it with them afterwards. Doing it this way would not be legal, and indeed we did prove to have huge difficulties later with the management committee, who wanted to throw us out into the street, but we overcame them in the end and managed to stay. The flat was lovely, just what we wanted. It had three bedrooms, and a huge living room at the front from which you could see the river. So that problem was solved, and Sophie was delighted, as we would be so close to Lower Mall. We all looked forward to visiting each other and to enjoyable walks along the towpath.

Having succeeded in my quest, which took most of February, I collapsed. It had been a stressful month: first my father's death, then not only the house hunting but also the discovery that Min, who I loved so very much, was not going to be any help as far as financial and practical support was concerned. We were not even sure how we were going to pay the rent, though Sophie, generous as always, had come up with a deposit and the first month's payment. So I was anxious and stressed, and at the beginning of March I succumbed to a bad throat infection, with extreme pain and a fever, and was ordered to spend a few days in bed. Min was kind and helpful, looked after William and brought me endless cups of tea.

I was lying there feeling very sorry for myself when the phone rang. It was Percy. My mother had been taken ill at the film studios and was at home at Lower Mall, in bed. Could we get over to see her? Feeling too ill to move I sent Min over. He came back with bad news. Sophie was very ill indeed – the cancer had come back. Dr Henderson had her on morphine and a nurse was being hired to stay with her.

Next day I managed to get up and get over to Lower Mall, to find Sophie barely conscious. She believed she was dying and was worrying about having huge debts but everyone kept telling her she would be fine. Next day she was not conscious at all. The day after, Percy and I were in the sitting room while the nurse, an unpleasant and officious woman, fussed around doing something or other. Then the nurse came in and told us it was all over. Sophie had died. We went in to see her. My only thought was that this was not my mother: this tiny, empty shell lying on the bed. Sophie had gone.

Percy was upright and stoical, and I was strong and practical. Neither of us cried. I found a firm of funeral directors and asked them to arrange to come and take her away as soon as possible. Poor George Goetschius and Peter Gill, both devastated, were left alone in the house, and Donald Howarth, having just gone to his cottage in Wales, was summoned back to keep George company. Soon the funeral people came to take the body away. As there is no parking in front of the house they had to carry her along Lower Mall for quite a distance and as I was not there to see it I have always wondered exactly how they did so.

I went to the bank and told them she had died. It was here that I discovered her true age, which she had lied about for most of her life. I had thought she was fifty-nine but discovered that she was in fact sixty-five, having been born in 1900. I arranged the funeral. It had to be Golders Green again. So all of that was arranged, and this time we would have some hymns, which Sophie loved for all her doubts about organised religion.

I had not shed a tear. I was in shock but I did not realise this, just thinking I was being very practical. I went to the hairdressers to have my hair done for the funeral and right opposite the hairdressers was the very firm of undertakers who were looking after Sophie. Georgina was with me and I pointed to the place and said, 'They've got my mother in there', but it was not true as this was in Notting Hill and she was at their Kensington Branch.

I decided I did not want to wear black at the funeral: it was too depressing and I was sure Sophie would not like it. So I went to Biba and bought myself a new coat in a wonderful daffodil yellow. Money was not going to be a problem now as I would have Lower Mall, which I could let. Sophie was right and there were huge debts but they could be paid off and I would be able to pay the rent in Putney. Perhaps we could even think about getting a cottage in the country.

So, less than six weeks later, there we all were back at Golders Green. I smiled and smiled – everyone said how well I was taking it. In those days no one had heard of being in denial. Then it was back to life in Putney. I managed to get myself some work making props and masks for the Court and graduated soon afterwards to reading scripts for them and for Twentieth Century Fox, the income from which, together with the rent from Lower Mall, meant we lived quite comfortably. It was not until the following July, when we went for the weekend to a cottage in the middle of a wood in Gloucestershire that something gave way inside me and I finally started to cry for Sophie and George.

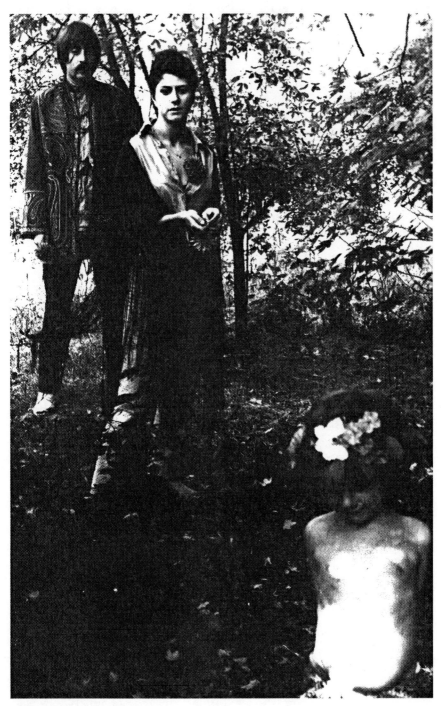

*Being flower children in a wood*

# POSTSCRIPT

Forty years have gone by since that dark year when I lost both my parents. Of course I have done a great many things since then, enough to fill another book. I made masks and props for a while, and spent a couple of years working as a script-reader. I was quite good at this, and Bill Gaskill employed me for a year as the Literary Manager of the Royal Court. Then I disappeared to a cottage in the wilds of Somerset where I lived for several years, wearing trailing garments, growing vegetables and eating brown rice. Sophie, who is Min's daughter, was born there, when William was six. Min and I never married, and we separated when Sophie was less than two. I married again, to a good kind man called Phil Jump, but eventually divorced from him too, though I have never been for any length of time without a relationship. I used to fall in love rather easily, but unfortunately out again as well. So all have been happy, but just have not lasted, though I have stayed friends with everyone I been involved with. There have been times in my life when I have thought that my father's defection had some bearing on my own attitude to relationships (drop them before they drop you, perhaps?), but I am not sure this is quite the answer. I have also thought that I might have been avoiding the kind of constant attachment that made my mother suffer so much, and certainly I still believe it better not to be too dependent on anyone else for one's own happiness. But there is another part of me that envies Sophie for being able to love the same person so much for so long. Also I have realised that my parents' relationship was astonishingly stable, given the level of infidelity and promiscuity practised by just about everyone else in their circle, and that is a source of admiration to me.

After I left Somerset I spent several years teaching meditation, mostly in Bristol. Then I finally decided to get myself a proper education, and, despite my lack of A-levels, talked myself onto a degree course in English Literature at North London Polytechnic. From there I went on to Oxford University as a postgraduate student, and spent several enjoyable years there, researching and teaching. Then I got a job at a small university college in Lancashire, and I have been there ever since, teaching and writing academic books.

It has always been a sadness to me that my children never had a chance to know their grandparents, who would, I know, have been proud of them. Both of them have gone into the theatre, William as an actor and Sophie as a stage designer. Percy, who lived to the great age of ninety five, was a wonderful support to us. Strong, independent and full of energy – she continued to go to work, at the theatre-design school she started, until about six months before she died – she loved my children and grandchildren deeply, and was unfailingly kind and generous to us all. We feel her absence very much.

And after all this time, I still miss my parents a great deal. It was many years – twenty at least – before I could speak of their deaths without physically shaking, I suppose from the effort of containing the emotion. But I don't want to suggest that my feelings about them were the same. For my mother I always felt sheer grief, a sense of regret and loss. She would have been so happy to see my children growing up, and how she would have loved my grandchildren, her great-grandchildren. I miss her warmth, her humour, her generosity. I know I was less close to her in the years before her death and that saddens me: writing about our relationship in her last few years has made me realise how much more I could have tried to share in her feelings, and indeed to involve her in mine. The smell of Marcel Rochas Femme, or the sound of a drawer sliding shut in her old chest of drawers, can bring her back to me with force, and probably always will.

With George it has been a different and a more complicated story. I had felt rejected by him since he left, and this was to continue for a long time. I have already written about my pain at seeing his will in black and white more than twenty years after his death. But over the years, and most recently this has increased, I have become aware of a powerful sense of unfinished business, a need to be reconciled. Images of fathers and daughters reunited can bring instant tears – Lear and Cordelia, Pericles and Marina, even the Railway Children: 'Daddy, oh my Daddy!'. I want him to reappear out of a cloud of steam, come walking down the platform into my arms. He won't, of course, he can't. And for a long time I thought he wouldn't want to. But my feelings about him have changed enormously since I started to think and to write about him – to figure him out. Reading his wartime letters told me that he loved me even before he met me, and I feel sure now that he went on loving me, even when shame and guilt made him strange and shy and awkward. Busy, often distant, emotionally confused, he managed despite everything to be what I now think of as a good father. My greatest sadness now is the knowledge of how proud he would have been of me if he could see me now, having finally found out that I can do something well and enjoy doing it.

Although I tried to follow in his footsteps by going into the theatre, they were the wrong kind of footsteps. But George was also a teacher and so I have followed him into that. People have commented, sometimes rather patronisingly, on his apparently simplistic style of teaching: how he would by saying 'There are three hundred and sixty five days in a year'. It was exciting to read that recently and to realise how remarkably similar his mind must have been to my own. If there is anything I have been committed to over the past few years both in teaching and in writing, it has been clarity of style and approach. So I love to read of his own obvious commitment to beginning with the basics and resolutely avoiding obfuscation.

My upbringing was certainly an unusual one, not only because of the milieu in which I grew up, but also because of the way in which my parents seem to have allowed me to make so many decisions about what I wanted to do with my life from an extremely early age. I wonder how deliberate and reasoned this approach was. It is interesting to reflect that George did consciously believe in it where his assistant directors at the Court – who were, after all, his surrogate children – were concerned:

> *I have never said 'No' to anyone. I have said, 'If you do this, that will happen: do you want that?'. If they insist, I allow them to have their way and take the consequences on my own shoulders. I think this is the best way to bring them up. If I say 'No' they will never be convinced that they were wrong and I was right.*

Although he never voiced this principle to me, looking back I can see that it did in fact inform his attitude to child-rearing to a large extent (he actually uses the term 'bring them up' in relation to the assistants). So although I have sometimes regretted that he was not more of a heavy father to me – insisting that I stay on at school and take my A-levels, for example – I do not regret the rather odd but distinctly enjoyable versions of my education, both in and out of school, that resulted from his refusal to insist. When I finally did get properly educated it was because I really wanted it myself.

So, looking back, I cannot really wish anything away. Of course I am extremely sorry that Sophie was so badly hurt by my father's departure. I could say I wish it had not had to happen, but the fact is that it did. I like to think that if she had had a few more years she might finally have come to terms with it, and built on the love and support of so many devoted people – Peter Gill, George Goetschius and others – with which she was surrounded in those last years, to make a strong and happy single life for herself. And I cannot begrudge George the great happiness he enjoyed with Jocelyn for such a relatively short time.

I started with a letter from my father and I will finish with one. Like many of his wartime letters, this one finds him musing on my future. He worries, as all good parents do, but he is clear sighted and pragmatic. And, although he had not yet met me, he got it pretty much right. The letter was written from 'somewhere between Rangoon and Columbo', as the ship bringing him home at the end of the war slowly made its way, 'cruising along on a beautiful deep blue sea with flying fish to watch'. He had been reading a book by Virginia Woolf, and reflecting on the extreme sensitivity that had led her to commit suicide in 1941:

*I sometimes wonder if we will do wrong to Harriet to teach her to know the finer sides of life and to be sensitive to artistic influences. Will we not thereby open her to more suffering in later life; it is a moot point. We have both of us seen enough during this war of the materialistic smash-and-grab attitude which is so acceptable in this modern world that we ought to be able to impart a deal of knowledge on these lines. And yet, of course, we cannot. She will just have to fight her own battle as we have done. She was born of us, and that can't be changed. She seems to have a deal of gaiety, and that should see her through, when she gets beyond the irresponsibility of youth.*

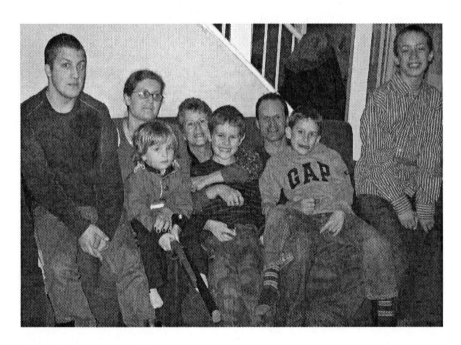

*Surrounded by my descendents:*
*Oli, Sophie, Cai, me, George, William, Ben and Jaz*

# INDEX

**Abbreviations**
ESC  English Stage Company
GD   George Devine
HD   Harriet Devine
SD   Sophie Devine

Numbers in italics refer to illustrations

# U
Ure, Mary, 83, 101, 102

# W
Warner, David, 145, *145*, 159
Warren, Iris, 136
Weigel, Helene, 164
Wesker, Arnold, 100, 101, 109, 111, 113-114, 115, *114*, 141
Wesker, Dusty, 101, *114*
Wilson, Angus, *79*, 80
Woolf, Leonard, 91
Woolf, Virginia, 91, 177
Wynne, David, 90

# Y
Yogi, Maharishi Mahesh, 136
Young, Jimmy, 160
Young, Wayland, 115

Printed in the United Kingdom
by Lightning Source UK Ltd.
109324UKS00001BA/67-141